ATLAS OF
INFECTIOUS DISEASES

ATLAS OF

INFECTIOUS DISEASES

David R. Stone, MD

Assistant Professor
Tufts University School of Medicine
Attending Physician
Divisions of Geographic Medicine and Infectious Diseases
New England Medical Center
and Department of Medicine
Lemuel Shattuck Hospital
Boston, Massachusetts

Sherwood L. Gorbach, MD

Professor of Community Health, Medicine, and Molecular Biology
Tufts University School of Medicine
Attending Physician
New England Medical Center and St. Elizabeth's Hospital
Boston, Massachusetts

W.B. SAUNDERS COMPANY
A *Harcourt Health Sciences Company*
Philadelphia London New York St. Louis Sydney Toronto

W.B. SAUNDERS COMPANY

A *Harcourt Health Sciences Company*

The Curtis Center
Independence Square West
Philadelphia, Pennsylvania 19106

Library of Congress Cataloging-in-Publication Data

Stone, David R.
    Atlas of infectious diseases / David R. Stone, Sherwood L. Gorbach.
— 1st ed.
        p.   cm.
    Includes bibliographical references.
    ISBN 0-7216-7032-6
    1. Communicable diseases Atlases.   2. Gorbach, Sherwood L.
    II. Title.
    [DNLM: 1. Communicable Diseases Atlases.   WC 17 S877a 2000]
RC113.2.S76   2000
616.9—DC21
DNLM/DLC   99-31874

ATLAS OF INFECTIOUS DISEASES   0-7216-7032-6

Printed in the United States of America

Last digit is the print number: 9   8   7   6   5   4   3   2

PREFACE

Establishing the diagnosis of infectious disease, perhaps more than any other pathologic entity in medicine, can be assisted enormously by a photograph. A characteristic skin lesion can implicate the causative microorganism even before a physical examination is performed or laboratory tests are obtained. Of course, the image is only helpful when the physician recognizes its true significance. The purpose of this *Atlas* is to provide pictures of disease entities that can be used by the astute clinician for early recognition of an underlying infection, whether localized or systemic. The accompanying tables and legends add some factual substance to the condition under consideration to help develop a differential diagnosis, order the appropriate confirmatory tests, and undertake appropriate treatment.

Susan Sontag wrote, "The camera makes everyone a tourist in other people's reality, and eventually in one's own." (*New York Review of Books,* 18 April 1974). Applied to medical diagnosis, the photographic image can transport the mind of the reader to the bedside, where he or she can be a silent player in the drama of the pathologic process. In this way the reader can visualize the subsequent enactments of diagnosis and treatment and make the image a part of his or her reality and memory bank. When the scene replays itself in real life by the appearance of a real patient, the physician can recall the image of the camera and translate it to a specific diagnosis.

In preparing this volume, we relied on our own clinical experience and our personal film collections. In addition, we are grateful to the following persons who made available to us with great generosity their experiences and photograph collections: Mary Anderson, Nicholas Blevins, Colin Carmody, Mark Drapkin, Jay Duker, David Hamer, Carl Heilman, Linden Hu, Michael Lew, Katherine McGowan, Sampson Munn, Athena Pappas, and David Wyler.

David R. Stone
Sherwood L. Gorbach

CONTENTS

1

HEAD AND NECK INFECTIONS

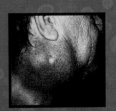
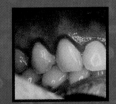
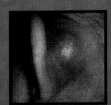

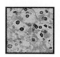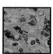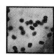

DEEP FASCIAL SPACE INFECTIONS

Soft tissue infections of the head and neck can have a dramatic appearance, with swelling and disfigurement. Signs of sepsis can develop rapidly. Spread through fascial planes can lead to serious complications when the infection is present around the great vessels or in the retropharyngeal space. Infection in the orbit can lead to vision loss as well as intracranial extension. It is paramount that the origin of the infection and the extent of spread be determined as quickly as possible so that surgical drainage and antibiotic therapy can be initiated rapidly.

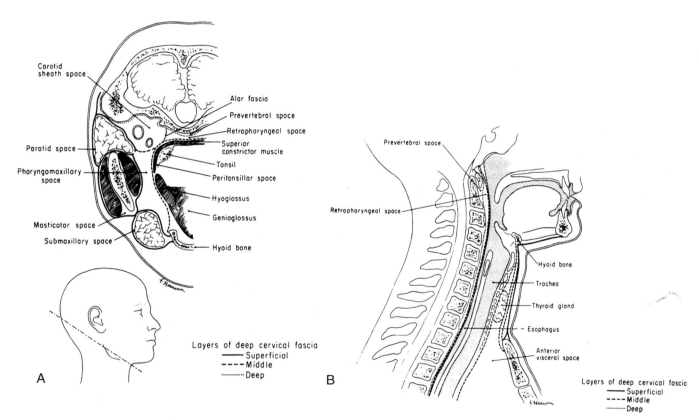

FIGURE 1–1

A, Midsagittal section of the neck illustrating anterior visceral, retropharyngeal, and prevertebral spaces. (From Levitt GW: Cervical fascia and deep neck infections. Laryngoscope 80:409–435, 1970.) **B,** Oblique section through the head. (From Langenbrunner DJ, Dajani S: Pharyngomaxillary space abscess with carotid artery erosion. Arch Otolaryngol 94:447–457, 1971. Copyright 1971, American Medical Association.)

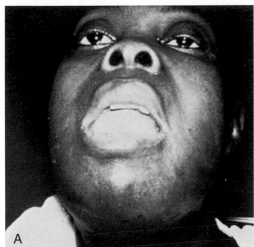

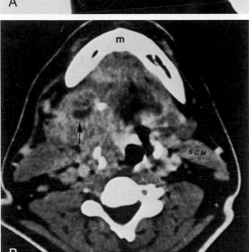

FIGURE 1–2

A, Patient with Ludwig's angina, revealing massive sublingual swelling, with upward protrusion of the tongue and bilateral neck swelling. **B,** Axial view CT scan of patient with Ludwig's angina revealing lucent zone *(arrow)* in submandibular space posterior to mylohyoid muscle. M, mandible; SCM, sternocleidomastoid. (Courtesy of Dr. A. Weber, Massachusetts Eye and Ear Infirmary, Boston, Massachusetts.)

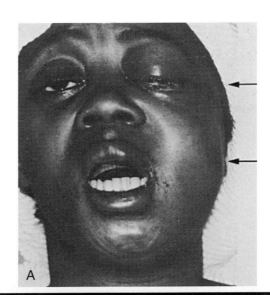

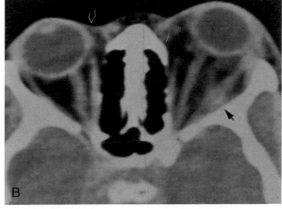

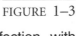

FIGURE 1–3

A, Pterygopalatine space and temporal space infection, with an orbital abscess in a patient with an upper molar tooth abscess. **B,** Extension of pterygopalatine space infection into the left orbit; soft tissue mass is evident *(arrow).* (Courtesy of Dr. A. Weber, Massachusetts Eye and Ear Infirmary, Boston, Massachusetts.)

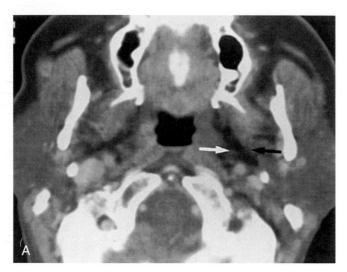

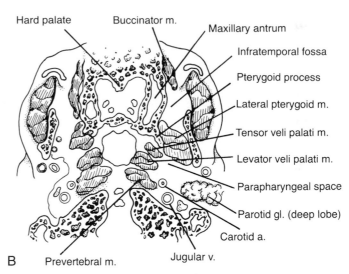

Hard palate   Buccinator m.
Maxillary antrum
Infratemporal fossa
Pterygoid process
Lateral pterygoid m.
Tensor veli palati m.
Levator veli palati m.
Parapharyngeal space
Parotid gl. (deep lobe)
Carotid a.
Prevertebral m.   Jugular v.

FIGURE 1–4

A, Parapharyngeal space (CT). **B,** Parapharyngeal space (anatomy). The triad of (1) tonsillar prolapse and swelling of the lateral pharyngeal wall, (2) trismus, and (3) parotid swelling indicates an abscess in the parapharyngeal space.

FIGURE 1–5

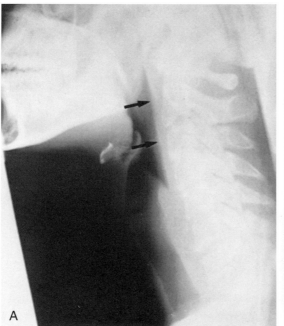

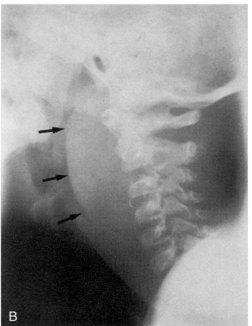

Retropharyngeal space. **A,** Normal lateral cervical view. **B,** Expansion of prevertebral soft tissues by retropharyngeal abscess. (Courtesy of Dr. A. Weber, Massachusetts Eye and Ear Infirmary, Boston, Massachusetts.)

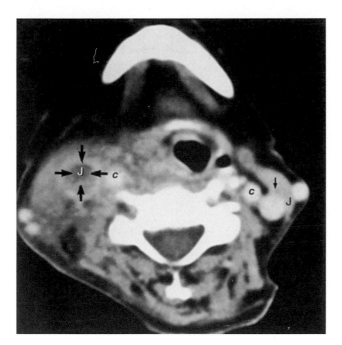

FIGURE 1–6

Jugular venous thrombosis. Contrast-enhanced axial CT scan at C3 shows the normal left carotid *(c)* and jugular *(J)* vessels *(arrow).* The right common carotid is normal *(arrow),* but the jugular vein is enlarged with a dense or enhancing wall *(arrows)* surrounding the more lucent intraluminal clot. Lemierre's disease, which often is caused by *Fusobacterium necrophorum,* is associated with jugular venous thrombosis and sepsis. (Courtesy of Dr. A. Weber, Massachusetts Eye and Ear Infirmary, Boston, Massachusetts.)

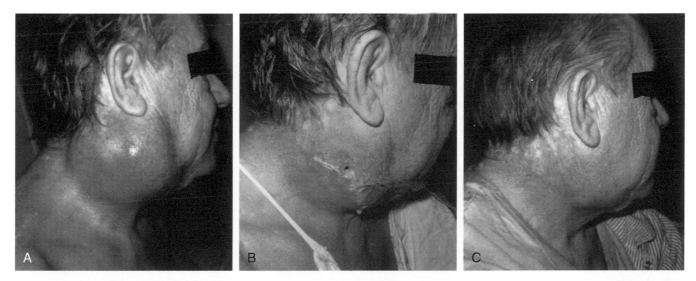

Cervicofacial actinomycosis with a large mass at the angle of the jaw. **A,** Initial presentation as a large fluctuant mass. **B,** Later in the course with induration and a sinus tract. **C,** The lesion after a 6-month course of penicillin.

FIGURE 1–7

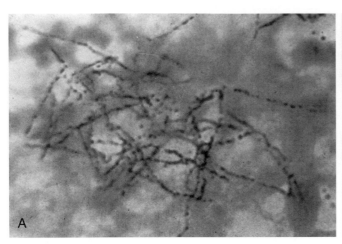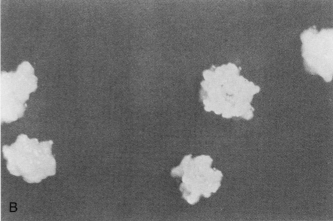

FIGURE 1–8

A, Gram stain appearance of agents of actinomycosis: branching "beaded" gram-positive bacilli. **B,** Colonies of *Actinomyces israelii* showing the molar tooth appearance.

EPIGLOTTITIS AND CROUP

With the advent of the *Haemophilus influenzae* type b vaccine, the incidence of epiglottitis has diminished in the pediatric population. Recognition of the symptoms and signs of epiglottitis and confirmation via lateral neck films are crucial in an emergency room setting. In addition to *H. influenzae,* other pathogens such as *Streptococcus pneumoniae, Staphylococcus aureus,* group A *Streptococcus,* and *Haemophilus parainfluenzae* are occasionally responsible.

FIGURE 1–9

Epiglottitis. Lateral neck films of adults with epiglottitis. Patient in **A** had no microbiological diagnosis. **B,** Culture from this patient grew *H. influenzae* type b. Note in each of the radiographs the edematous epiglottis, which produces the so called thumb sign. (*B* courtesy of Dr. Mark Drapkin, Newton Wellesley Hospital, Newton, Massachusetts.)

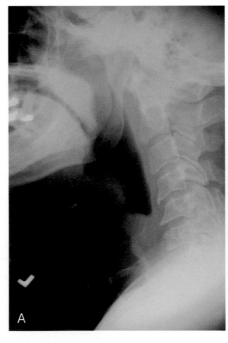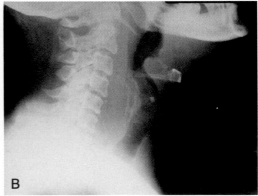

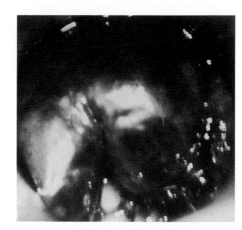

FIGURE 1–10

Epiglottitis. View from the pharynx showing intense inflammation and swelling of the epiglottis. It is imperative that the epiglottis be visualized only after the airway is secured by intubation or tracheostomy.

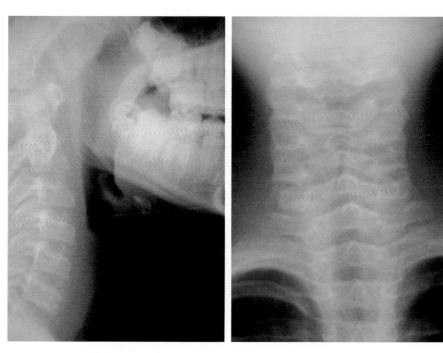

FIGURE 1–11

Croup. The epiglottis is normal size. On the posteroanterior film, subglottic stenosis can be seen.

FIGURE 1–12

Croup. Inflammation of the subglottic region has significantly reduced the diameter of the airway. Parainfluenza virus is the most common cause of croup.

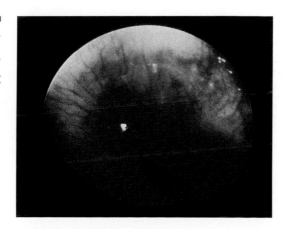

ORAL CAVITY AND PHARYNX

The oral cavity and the pharynx are affected by various organisms, often bacterial and viral in origin. Most infections are painful and thus are brought to medical attention early.

FIGURE 1–13

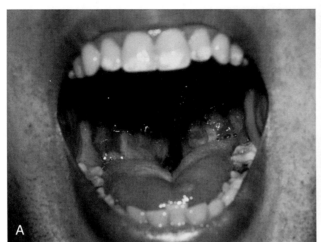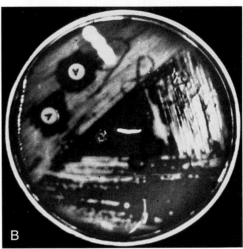

A, Patient with group A streptococcal pharyngitis. **B,** Throat culture from patient in *A,* showing colonies of β-hemolytic streptococci growing on sheep's blood agar. Bacitracin disks (marked A) show zone of inhibition of growth.

FIGURE 1–14

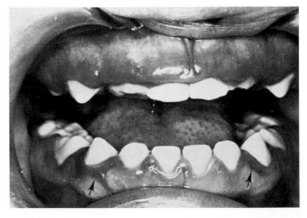

Acute herpetic gingivostomatitis: gingivitis. This child's gums are tender, swollen, and hyperemic. There is a bright red line *(arrows)* along the dental margin. (From Oxman MN: Herpes stomatitis. *In* Braude AI, Davis CE, Fierer J [eds]: Infectious Diseases and Medical Microbiology, ed 2. Philadelphia, WB Saunders, 1986, pp 752–772.)

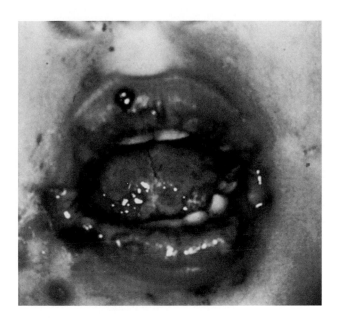

FIGURE 1–15

Acute herpetic gingivostomatitis. In addition to having vesicles on the oral mucosa, palate, and tongue, this child has herpetic vesicles on the lips and perioral skin. (From Oxman MN: Herpes stomatitis. *In* Braude AI, Davis CE, Fierer J [eds]: Infectious Diseases and Medical Microbiology, ed 2. Philadelphia, WB Saunders, 1986, pp 752–772.)

FIGURE 1–16

Herpes simplex virus (HSV). Multiple, painful, ulcerative lesions occur in primary HSV infections. Although most oral lesions are caused by HSV-1, HSV-2 can be cultured sporadically from such lesions.

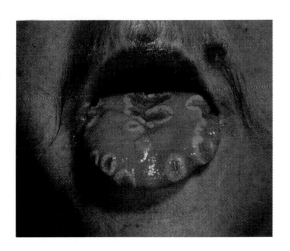

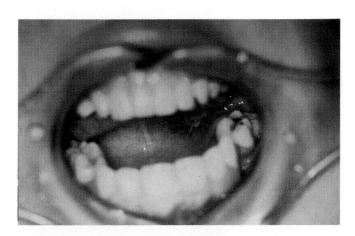

FIGURE 1–17

Varicella-zoster virus (VZV). Unilateral pharyngitis can be a manifestation of VZV reactivation. The painful blisters may resemble herpangina. The lesions are unilateral. Reactivation emanates from the geniculate ganglion. A positive culture is the gold standard for diagnosing herpetic infections.

FIGURE 1–18

Ramsay Hunt syndrome. Unilateral cranial nerve (CN) VII palsy may be a manifestation of the Ramsay Hunt syndrome, which is caused by a reactivation of VZV, either in the ear or in the posterior pharynx (CN VII or IX).

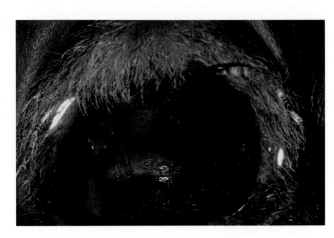

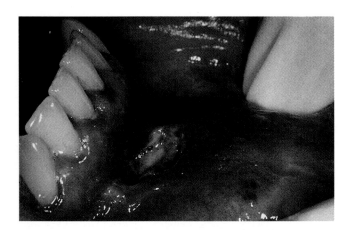

FIGURE 1–19

Aphthous ulcer. Aphthous ulcers may recur and often resemble HSV infection. (Courtesy of Dr. Athena Pappas, Tufts University School of Dental Medicine, Boston, Massachusetts.)

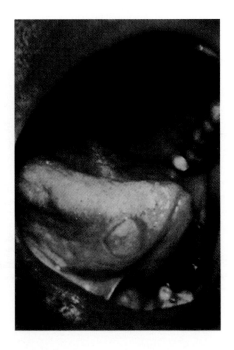

FIGURE 1–20

Syphilis is always in the differential diagnosis of an ulcerative lesion in the oropharynx. This large chancre was painless.

TABLE 1–1

Differences Between Herpes Simplex Virus Types 1 and 2

CHARACTERISTICS	HSV-1	HSV-2	CHARACTERISTICS	HSV-1	HSV-2
Clinical			**Latency**		
Manifestations of primary infection			In trigeminal and cervical sensory ganglia	+	–
Acute herpetic gingivostomatitis	+*	–†	In sacral sensory ganglia	–	+
Acute herpetic pharyngotonsillitis	+	–‡	Frequency of recurrence when latent in trigeminal and cervical sensory ganglia	+	–
Acute herpetic keratoconjunctivitis	+	–	Frequency of recurrence when latent in sacral sensory ganglia	–	+
Neonatal herpes simplex infections	±§	+			
Manifestations of recurrent infection			**Biochemical**		
Herpes labialis	+	–	DNA guanine + cytosine	68%	69%
Herpes keratitis	+	–	Homology between viral DNAs		Approximately 50%
Manifestations of primary or recurrent infection			Stability of virus-specific thymidine kinase at 40°C	+	–
Cutaneous herpes					
Skin above the waist	+	–	**Biology**		
Skin below the waist	–	+	Neurotropism in mice on peripheral inoculation	Less neuro-tropic	More neuro-tropic
Hands or arms	+	+	Pock size on chick chorioallantoic membrane	Small	Large
Herpetic whitlow	+	+	Plaque formation in chick embryo cell monolayer culture	–	+
Eczema herpeticum	+	–			
Herpes genitalis	±‖	+	Temperature sensitivity of replication (40°C)	–	+
Herpes simplex encephalitis	+	–	Inhibition of replication by heparin, neomycin, polylysine	+	–
Herpes simplex meningitis	±¶	+			
Disseminated HSV infection in immuno-compromised patients	+	+	Inhibition of replication by thymidine	–	+
Epidemiologic					
Transmission	Nonsexual	Sexual			
Epidemiologic association with carcinoma of the cervix	–	+			

HSV-1 and HSV-2 can be differentiated unequivocally by serologic techniques, by DNA-to-DNA hybridization, by restriction endonuclease fingerprinting of viral DNA, and by electrophoretic analysis of virus-specified proteins. ■

*+, Frequent or predominant cause, or significantly greater than the other serotype.
†–, Infrequent cause (except under special epidemiologic circumstances), or significantly less or lower than the other serotype.
‡HSV-2 is frequently isolated when pharyngotonsillitis is associated with orogenital sexual contact.
§HSV-1 is isolated from approximately 30% of cases, reflecting the increasing frequency with which HSV-1 causes genital herpes (in the mother) as well as some cases of infection acquired postnatally from individuals shedding HSV-1.
‖HSV-1 is now being isolated from 10% to 40% of patients with primary genital herpes, reflecting the growing proportion of the population that is reaching the age of sexual activity without having experienced orolabial HSV-1 infection and the prevalence of orogenital sexual contact. Herpetic vulvovaginitis in infants is generally caused by HSV-1, acquired from adults or by autoinoculation of infected saliva.
¶ Some cases reported, but insufficient data to estimate frequency.
Modified from Oxman MN: Herpes stomatis. *In* Braude AI (ed): Infectious Diseases and Medical Microbiology, ed 2. Philadelphia, WB Saunders, 1986.

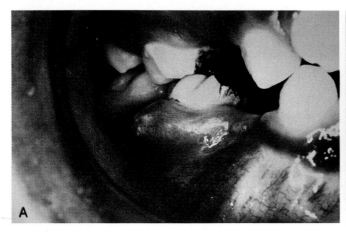 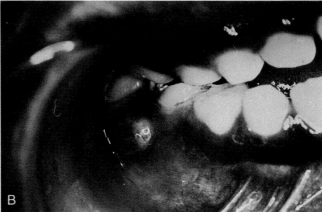

FIGURE 1–21   Abscessed tooth. Apical tooth abscess pointing through the alveolar bone.

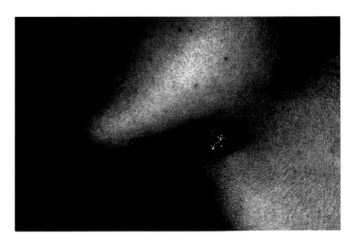

FIGURE 1–22

A cutaneous fistula to the neck has developed from an apical tooth abscess. This manifestation is rare today because of antibiotics and the access most patients have to emergency dental care.

FIGURE 1–23

Gingivitis. This patient has HIV infection. Note the areas of erythema in the gingiva. Patients usually experience bleeding gums after minimal trauma such as brushing the teeth. (Courtesy of Dr. Athena Pappas, Tufts University School of Dental Medicine, Boston, Massachusetts.)

TABLE 1–2

Relationship Between Clinical Forms of Periodontal Disease and Various Bacterial Species

CLINICAL ENTITY	BACTERIAL FACTOR
Gingivitis	
Experimental	Plaque accumulation streptococci, actinomycetes
Pregnancy	*Prevotella intermedia*
Puberty	*P. intermedia?*
Stress (acute necrotizing ulcerative gingivitis)	*P. intermedia,* spirochetes
Simple	Plaque accumulation, spirochetes
Generalized severe	Spirochetes
Periodontitis	
Prepuberty	Spirochetes, black-pigmented species
Localized juvenile	*Actinobacillus actinomycetemcomitans*
Early onset	Spirochetes, *Porphyromonas gingivalis, A. actinomycetemcomitans*
Adult	Spirochetes, black-pigmented species, *A. actinomycetemcomitans*
Progressive	*Bacteroides forsythus, Campylobacter rectus* (formerly *Wolinella recta*)

CERVICAL ADENITIS

Many infections in the head and neck can spread to the regional cervical lymph nodes. Historically, mycobacterial infections, both typical and atypical strains, have been the most common causes of chronic unilateral cervical adenitis. Many of these infections require surgical excision.

FIGURE 1–24

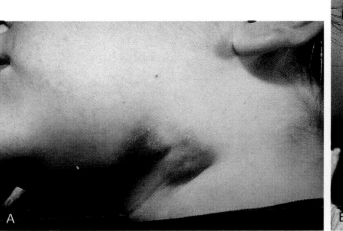
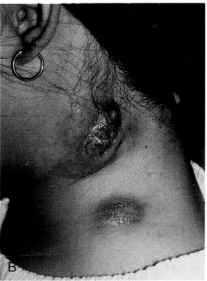

Scrofula. **A,** Cervical swelling caused by an atypical mycobacterial infection of anterior cervical lymph nodes is seen in this child. **B,** Chronic drainage from an infected lymph node. *Mycobacterium tuberculosis* was cultured from this lesion.

FIGURE 1–25

This 3-year-old child from the Midwest presented with the ulceroglandular syndrome of tularemia. Without treatment, fistulae may develop and drain for months.

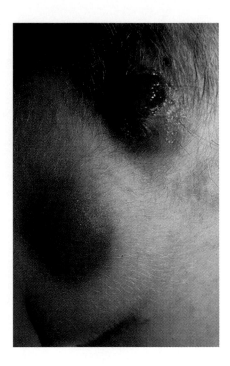

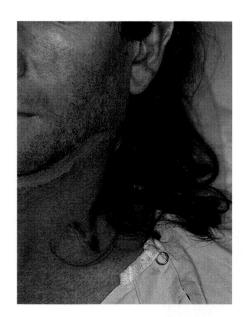

FIGURE 1–26

Staphylococcal lymphadenitis. Because of prior skin grafting, this patient was prone to recurrent facial cellulitis due to *Staphylococcus aureus.* Enlargement and tenderness in the cervical lymph nodes was marked weeks after the acute cellulitis had resolved.

INFECTIONS IN IMMUNOCOMPROMISED HOSTS

Patients with an altered immune system can experience manifestations of infections in the head and neck region. (There is a section on head and neck manifestations of HIV infection in Chapter 6.) Diseases in neutropenic patients, transplant patients, and diabetics are usually severe. Invasive fungal infections are often life threatening and are associated with high morbidity and mortality rates.

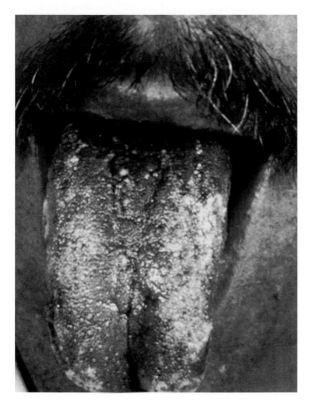

FIGURE 1–27

Candidiasis. Whitish, curdlike exudates present on mucous membranes that are easily scraped off with a tongue depressor are characteristic of candidiasis. This is often associated with candidal esophagitis, which may result in severe dysphagia.

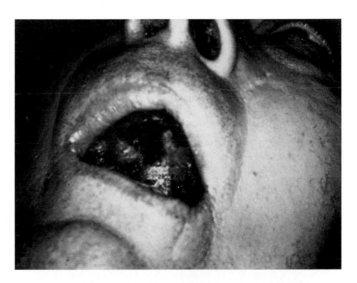

FIGURE 1–28

Necrosis of the hard palate due to invasion by *Rhizopus* species in a renal transplant patient taking corticosteroids.

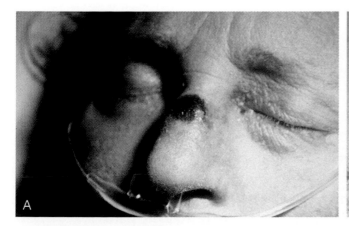 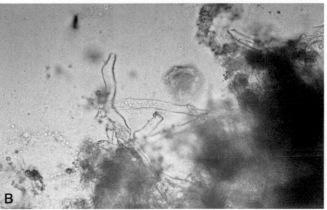

Rhizopus. This patient had diabetes and renal failure and was on dialysis. A necrotizing fungal infection that developed throughout the nasal cavity grew *Rhizopus.*

FIGURE 1–29

FUNGAL

Coccidioides immitis infections of the nose are common and most likely represent both primary inoculation and disseminated disease. When lesions are present on the nose or upper lip, *Coccidioides* meningitis should be suspected.

FIGURE 1–30

This map displays the regions in which coccidioidomycosis is most highly endemic. The stippled areas represent the uncertain boundaries. (From Pappagianis D. *In* Stevens DA [ed]: Coccidioidomycosis. New York, Plenum Publishing, 1980, p 64.)

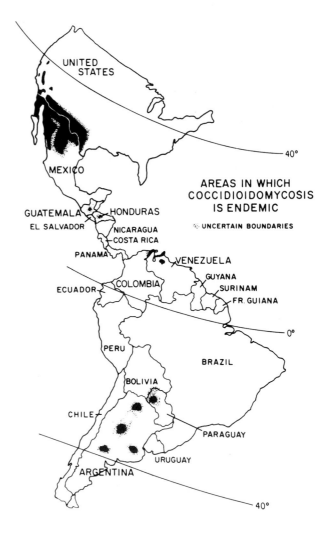

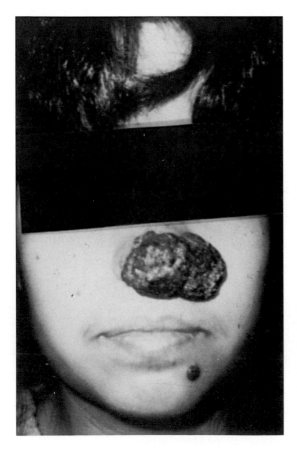

FIGURE 1–31

Two skin lesions on the face of a child with disseminated coccidioidomycosis: an exuberant verrucous, tumorlike lesion of the nose and one of the chin that appears nodular and granulomatous. (Courtesy of Dr. Richard Tucker, Wenatchee Valley Clinic, Wenatchee, Washington.)

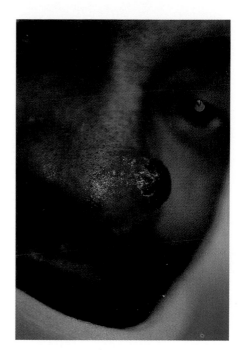

FIGURE 1-32

Coccidioides. Papular lesions may be an early manifestation of dis-seminated cocci.

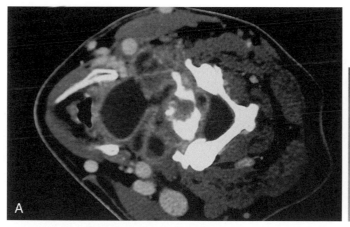

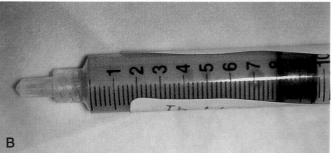

Coccidioides. This patient had disseminated disease. A submandibular ab-scess was drained and grew *Coccidioides immitis.*

FIGURE 1-33

OTITIS

Ear infections are common in clinical practice. Malignant otitis externa requires early diagnosis so that antibiotics can be initiated. Otologic examinations looking for occult sites of infection, especially in immunocompromised persons, must be routinely performed.

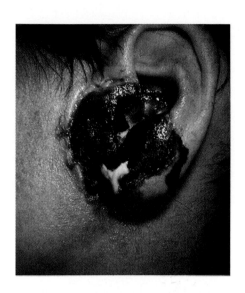

FIGURE 1–34

Malignant otitis externa. Typical appearance of late stage disease. Areas of necrosis are present. This patient had a *Pseudomonas aeruginosa* infection. (Courtesy of Dr. Mark Drapkin, Newton Wellesley Hospital, Newton, Massachusetts.)

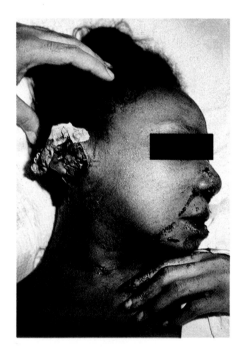

FIGURE 1–35

Otitis externa. This diabetic woman presented with malignant otitis externa. Cultures subsequently grew *Staphylococcus aureus*. Most cases are associated with *Pseudomonas*.

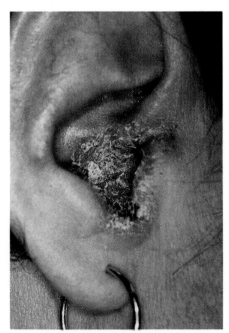

FIGURE 1–36

Chronic otitis externa. Chronic drainage and a crusty appearance are noted in this patient with chronic otitis externa. This patient had chronic drainage from the middle ear. (Courtesy of Dr. N. Blevins, New England Medical Center, Boston, Massachusetts.)

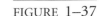

FIGURE 1–37

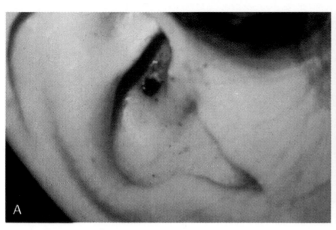
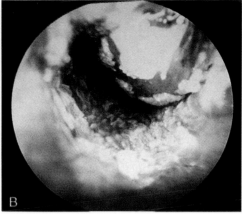

Otic herpes zoster. Lesions may be hard to find and must be distinguished from external otitis. Otic zoster can be associated with loss of taste in the anterior portion of the tongue and a facial palsy (Ramsay-Hunt syndrome).

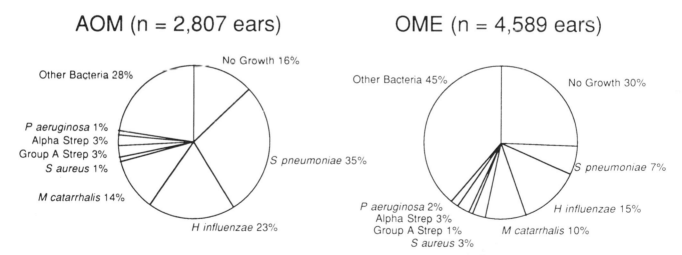

AOM (n = 2,807 ears)

No Growth 16%
Other Bacteria 28%
P aeruginosa 1%
Alpha Strep 3%
Group A Strep 3%
S aureus 1%
M catarrhalis 14%
S pneumoniae 35%
H influenzae 23%

OME (n = 4,589 ears)

Other Bacteria 45%
No Growth 30%
P aeruginosa 2%
Alpha Strep 3%
Group A Strep 1%
S aureus 3%
S pneumoniae 7%
H influenzae 15%
M catarrhalis 10%

Comparison of bacteria from middle-ear aspirates obtained by tympanocentesis in infants and children with acute otitis media (AOM) or otitis media with effusion (OME), the latter immediately before insertion of tympanostomy tubes. Totals may add up to more than 100% because of the presence of multiple pathogens. (From Bluestone CD, Stephenson JS, Martin LM: Ten-year review of otitis media pathogens. Pediatr Infect Dis J 11:S7–S11, 1992.)

FIGURE 1–38

FIGURE 1–39

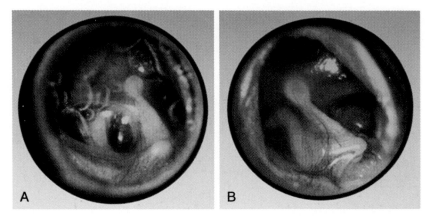

Serous otitis media. **A,** Fluid behind the tympanic membrane is noted. This often follows a viral infection in which there is transient blockage of the eustachian tube. The inner ear can become infected with bacteria. **B,** Negative pressure that occurs with a blockage of the eustachian tube leads to retraction of the tympanic membrane and accumulation of serous fluid. (Courtesy of Dr. N. Blevins, New England Medical Center, Boston, Massachusetts.)

FIGURE 1–40

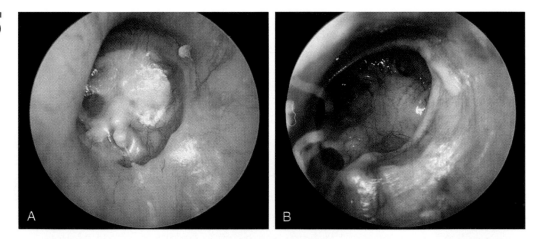

A, Myringitis. Acute bacterial otitis media leads to edema, erythema, and purulence of the tympanic membrane. The organisms most commonly causing the infection include *Streptococcus pneumoniae* and *H. influenzae.* **B,** Myringitis with perforation. (Courtesy of Dr. N. Blevins, New England Medical Center, Boston, Massachusetts.)

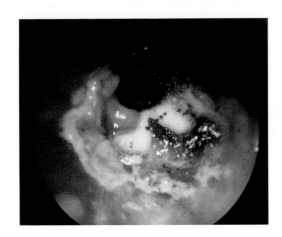

FIGURE 1–41

Fungal external otitis. *Aspergillus* spp. are often cultured in this localized infection. (Courtesy of Dr. N. Blevins, New England Medical Center, Boston, Massachusetts.)

SINUSITIS

TABLE 1–3

Microbial Causes of Acute Maxillary Sinusitis

	PREVALENCE MEAN (RANGE)	
MICROBIAL AGENT	Adults (%)	Children (%)
Bacteria		
Streptococcus pneumoniae	31 (20–35)	36
Haemophilus influenzae (nonencapsulated)	21 (6–26)	23
S. pneumoniae and *H. influenzae*	5 (1–9)	—
Anaerobes *(Bacteroides, Fusobacterium, Peptostreptococcus, Veillonella)*	6 (0–10)	—
Staphylococcus aureus	4 (0–8)	—
Streptococcus pyogenes	2 (1–3)	2
Branhamella (Moraxella) catarrhalis	2	19
Gram-negative bacteria	9 (0–24)	2
Viruses		
Rhinovirus	15	—
Influenza virus	5	—
Parainfluenza virus	3	2
Adenovirus	—	2

Adapted from Gwaltney JM Jr: Sinusitis. *In* Mandell GL, Douglas RG Jr, Bennett JE (eds): Principles and Practice of Infectious Diseases, ed 3. Churchill Livingstone, New York, 1990.

TABLE 1–4

The Clinical Spectrum and Investigation of Intracranial Complications of Sinusitis*

COMPLICATION	CLINICAL SIGNS	CEREBROSPINAL FLUID FINDINGS	COMPUTED TOMOGRAPHY	
			Plain	Contrast Enhanced
Meningitis	Headache, fever ++ Stiff neck, lethargy ++ Rapid death ++	High PMN count and protein; low glucose	Normal	Diffusely enhanced
Osteomyelitis	Pott puffy tumor ±	Normal	Bone defect	Bone defect
Epidural abscess or mucocele	Headache ± Fever ±	Normal	Lucent area	Biconvex capsule
Subdural empyema	Headache ++ Convulsions ++ Hemiplegia ++ Rapid death ++	High PMN count and protein; normal glucose	Lucent area	Crescent-shaped enhancement
Cerebral abscess	Convulsions + Headache + Personality change +	Lymphocytosis; normal glucose	Lucency with mass effect	Capsule
Venous sinus thrombosis (cavernous)	"Picket-fence" fever ++ Rapid death ++ (orbital edema ++, ocular palsies ++)	Normal or high PMN count	Nonspecific	Enhancing lesion

*±, May or may not be seen; +, seen frequently; ++ seen characteristically; PMN, polymorphonuclear leukocyte.
Modified from Fairbanks DNF, Milmoe GJ: Complications and sequelae—An otolaryngologist's perspective. Pediatr Infect Dis 4(Suppl 6):S75, 1985.

FIGURE 1–42

Anatomy of paranasal sinuses. The frontal, anterior ethmoidal, and maxillary sinuses drain into the middle meatus; the posterior ethmoidal and sphenoidal sinuses open into the superior meatus. Note that the ostium of the maxillary sinus drains at an obtuse angle toward the roof. The floor of the maxillary sinus is close to the superior alveolar ridge.

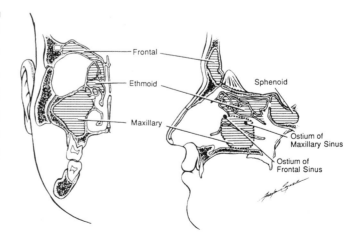

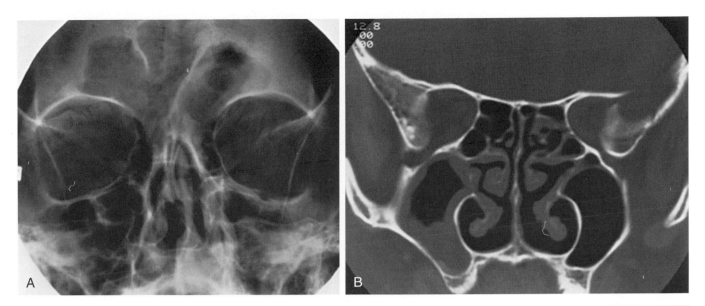

Radiographic studies of sinusitis. **A,** Caldwell view of the frontal and ethmoidal sinuses. Note partial opacification of both frontal sinuses with mucosal thickening in the left frontal sinus and associated sclerosis in the left
frontal bone. **B,** Coronal CT view of the ethmoidal and maxillary sinuses.
Note mucosal thickening in the right maxillary sinus. (*A* and *B* courtesy of
Dr. W. D. Robertson.)

FIGURE 1–43

FIGURE 1–44

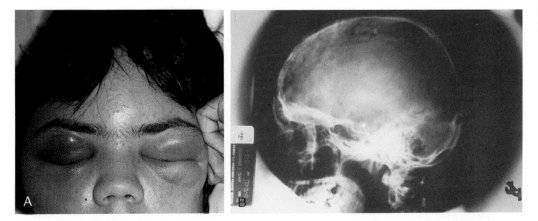

Frontal sinusitis. **A,** Infection of the frontal sinus has led to osteomyelitis of
the frontal bone. **B,** Subsequent swelling in the forehead is known as Pott's
puffy tumor. Osteomyelitis of the frontal bone is a rare complication of
frontal sinusitis.

FIGURE 1–45

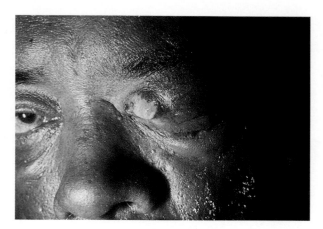

Frontal sinusitis with drainage. Spontaneous drainage from an infected frontal sinus was more common prior to the introduction of antibiotics.

FIGURE 1–46

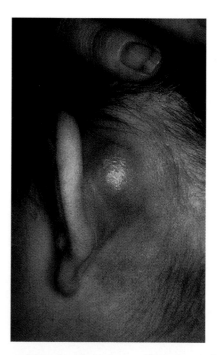

Mastoiditis. Swelling and tenderness over the mastoid bone is diagnostic for acute mastoiditis. Most common causes are *S. pneumoniae* and *H. influenzae*. (Courtesy of Dr. N. Blevins, New England Medical Center, Boston, Massachusetts.)

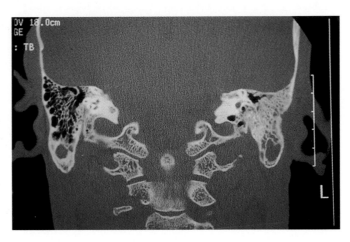

FIGURE 1–47

Mastoiditis x-ray film. Opacification of the mastoid air cells is visible on the left side of this coronal scan. (Courtesy of Dr. N. Blevins, New England Medical Center, Boston, Massachusetts.)

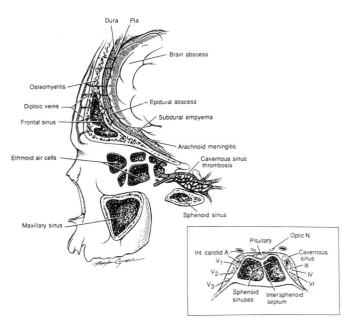

FIGURE 1–48

Intracranial complications of sinusitis. The sagittal section shows the major routes for intracranial extension of infection either directly or by the vascular supply. Note the proximity of the diploic veins to the frontal sinus and of the cavernous sinuses to the sphenoidal sinus. The coronal section demonstrates the structures adjoining the sphenoidal sinus.

FIGURE 1–49

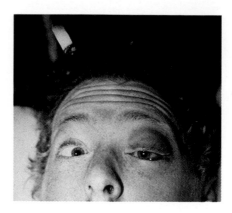

Cavernous sinus thrombosis. CN VI palsy leads to the inability to abduct the left eye past the midposition.

FIGURE 1–50

Cavernous sinus thrombosis.

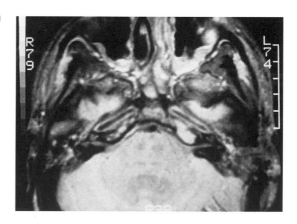

2

PULMONARY INFECTIONS

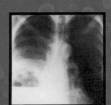
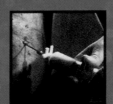
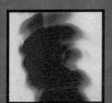

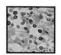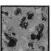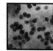

Infection of the lung is the leading cause of infectious mortality in the United States. Often a particular pathogen will produce a characteristic radiographic pattern. It is critical to obtain a good history of exposures and past medical problems for every patient with pneumonia. In addition, sputum evaluation is crucial in determining the most likely organism and directing appropriate antibiotics to treat that organism.

This chapter is divided into bacterial and fungal pneumonias. (Sections in the AIDS chapter and mycobacteria chapter are devoted to pulmonary infections as well.)

BACTERIAL PNEUMONIAS

TABLE 2–1

Chest Radiography: Differential Diagnosis

IMMUNOCOMPETENT	IMMUNOSUPPRESSED (ACQUIRED IMMUNODEFICIENCY SYNDROME)
Focal Opacity	**Focal Opacity**
Streptococcus pneumoniae	Pyogenic bacteria (as with immunocompetent)
Haemophilus influenzae	*Cryptococcus neoformans*
Mycoplasma pneumoniae	*Nocardia*
Legionella	*Mycobacterium tuberculosis*
Chlamydia pneumoniae	Kaposi's sarcoma
Staphylococcus aureus	
Mycobacterium tuberculosis	
Gram-negative bacteria	
Anaerobes	
Interstitial-Miliary	**Interstitial-Miliary**
Viruses	*Pneumocystis carinii*
Mycoplasma pneumoniae	*Mycobacterium tuberculosis*
Mycobacterium tuberculosis	Pathogenic fungi*
Pathogenic fungi*	*Leishmania donovani*
	Cytomegalovirus
Hilar Adenopathy ± Infiltrate	**Hilar Adenopathy**
Epstein-Barr virus	*Mycobacterium tuberculosis*
Francisella tularensis	*Cryptococcus neoformans*
Chlamydia psittaci	Pathogenic fungi*
Mycoplasma pneumoniae	Lymphoma
Mycobacterium tuberculosis	Kaposi's sarcoma
Pathogenic fungi*	
Atypical rubella	
Cavitation	**Cavitation**
Anaerobes	Gram-negative bacilli
Mycobacterium tuberculosis	*Mycobacterium tuberculosis*
Pathogenic fungi*	*Mycobacterium kansasii*
Gram-negative bacilli	*Cryptococcus neoformans*
Staphylococcus aureus	Pathogenic fungi*
	Rhodococcus equi
	Staphylococcus aureus (injection drug use) ■

*Pathogenic fungi: *Histoplasma capsulatum*, *Coccidioides immitis*, and *Blastomyces dermatitidis*.

TABLE 2–2

Bacteriology of Community-Acquired Pneumonia: Metaanalysis of 59 Reports, 1966 to 1995*

Total number of cases with bacterial pathogen	6104
Streptococcus pneumoniae	4432 (73%)
Haemophilus influenzae	833 (14%)
Legionella	272 (4%)
Staphylococcus aureus	157 (3%)
Gram-negative bacilli	103 (2%)
Klebsiella	56
Pseudomonas aeruginosa	18

*Analysis restricted to cases with a bacterial pathogen. No likely etiologic agent was detected in 11,229 cases.

Data from Fine MJ, Smith MA, Carson CA, et al: Prognosis and outcomes of patients with community-acquired pneumonia: A meta-analysis. JAMA 275:134–141, 1996.

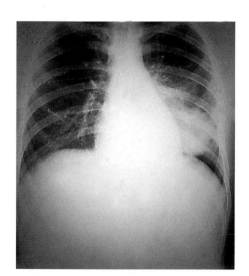

FIGURE 2–1

Nineteen-year-old male with pneumococcal pneumonia.

FIGURE 2–2

Typical colonies of *Streptococcus pneumoniae* on the surface of a blood agar plate. Central autolysis gives the colony the appearance of a checker (× 18). (Reproduced from *The Journal of Experimental Medicine,* 1953, vol 98, pp 21–34, by copyright permission of The Rockefeller University Press.)

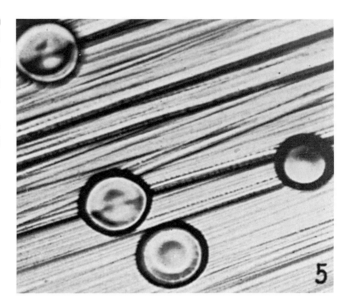

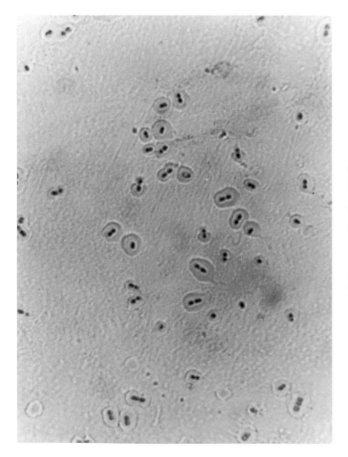

FIGURE 2–3

Quellung preparation of pneumococcal cells shows the refractile halo surrounding the bacterial cell (× 1100). (Reproduced from *The Journal of Experimental Medicine,* 1953, vol 98, pp 21–34, by copyright permission of The Rockefeller University Press.)

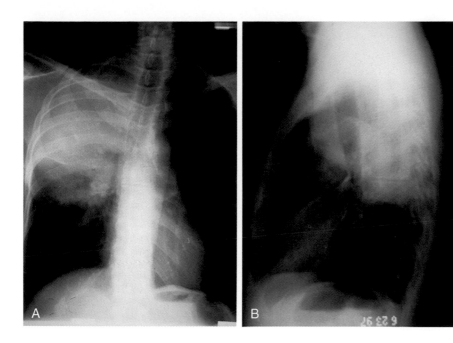

FIGURE 2–4

Klebsiella pneumoniae. **A,** Anterior view. **B,** Lateral view.

FIGURE 2–5

This patient has necrotizing pneumonia due to *K. pneumoniae.*

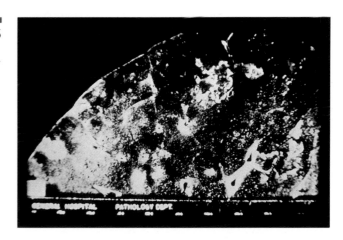

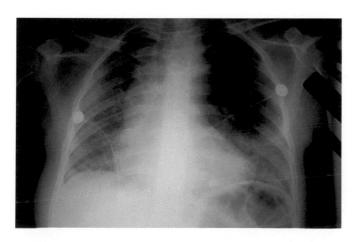

FIGURE 2–6

Pseudomonas pneumoniae.

FIGURE 2–7

This patient died of pneumonia caused by *Pseudomonas aeruginosa.* Extensive hemorrhage is seen.

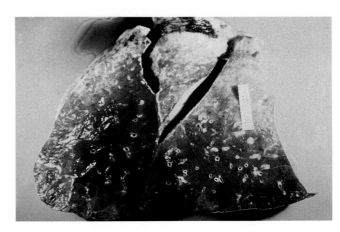

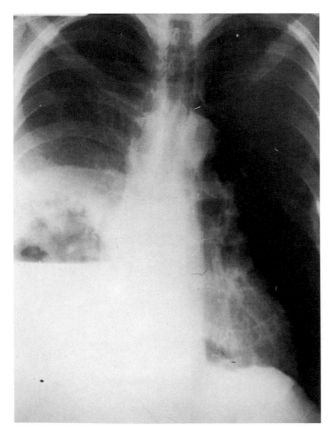

FIGURE 2–8

Chest radiograph of a patient showing a large lung abscess in the right lower hemithorax that was caused by *Rhodococcus equi.*

TABLE 2–3

Clinical Aids to the Etiologic Diagnosis of Atypical Pneumonia Syndrome

PATHOGEN	SYMPTOMS	SIGNS	HISTORY	LABORATORY
Influenza virus	Myalgia, severe respiratory distress	ARD	Epidemic	$\downarrow$ Po$_2$
Respiratory syncytial virus	Wheezing, persistent cough	Bronchospasm	—	—
Hantavirus	Severe respiratory distress	ARDS	Exposure to rodents or their excreta	Hemoconcentration, $\uparrow$ LDH, $\downarrow$ platelets
Adenovirus	—	—	Military, school, AIDS, transplant	—
Cytomegalovirus	—	Retinitis, colitis	AIDS, transplant	—
Chlamydia psittaci	—	—	Bird exposure	—
Mycoplasma pneumoniae	Insidious onset, cough	Negative chest examination findings	School, military	Cold agglutinins
Pneumocystis carinii	—	—	AIDS risk activity	$\downarrow$ Po$_2$, $\uparrow$ LDH

ARDS, Adult respiratory distress syndrome; AIDS, acquired immunodeficiency syndrome; LDH, lactate dehydrogenase; Po$_2$, oxygen tension.

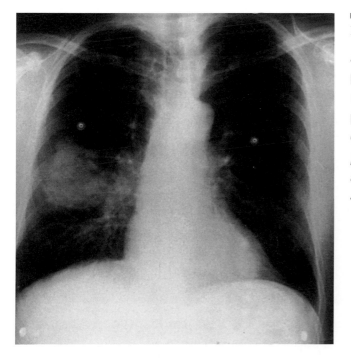

FIGURE 2–9

A 64-year-old smoker presented with fever and non-productive cough. The chest radiograph showed a rounded density in the right lower lobe. Malignant neoplasm was suspected. Culture of respiratory secretions obtained at bronchoscopy yielded *Legionella pneumophila.* (From Muder RR, Yu VL, Fang GD: Community-acquired Legionnaires' disease. Semin Respir Infect 4:32–39, 1989.)

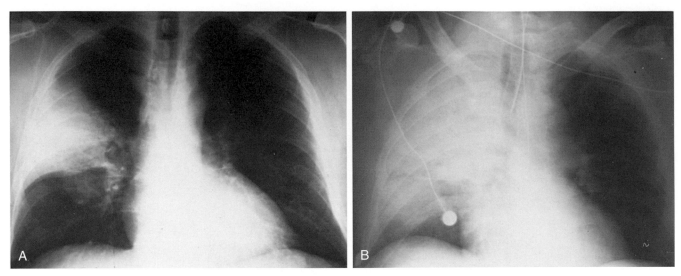

FIGURE 2–10

A 47-year-old man presented with chills and slightly productive cough. His history was remarkable only for cigarette smoking and essential hypertension. The chest radiograph showed a segmental infiltrate in the lower portion of the right upper lobe **(A).** Cephalosporin therapy was begun. By the third hospital day the infiltrate had progressed to the right upper lobe and the upper portion of the right lower lobe **(B).** Sputum culture obtained on admission yielded heavy growth of *L. pneumophila.* Erythromycin and rifampin were begun, followed by clinical response and ultimate recovery. (From Muder RR, Yu VL, Parry M: Radiology of *Legionella* pneumonia. Semin Respir Infect 2:242–254, 1987.)

FIGURE 2–11

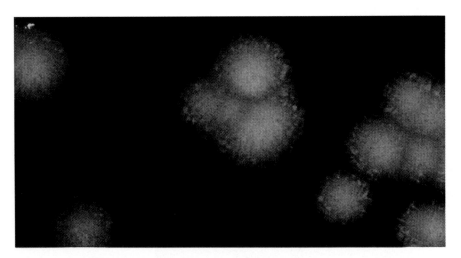

Colonies of *Legionella pneumophila* with characteristic ground-glass surface texture. (Magnification approximately × 10.)

TABLE 2–4

Epidemiologic and Clinical Characteristics of Respiratory Disease Caused by *Chlamydia*

FEATURE	C. PNEUMONIAE	C. TRACHOMATIS	C. PSITTACI
Natural host	Humans	Humans	Birds, mammals
Population	All ages	Infants, immunocompromised adults	Veterinarians, bird fanciers, poultry workers
Mode of transmission	Person to person: by aerosol droplets	Vertical: mother to infant	Bird to person: by aerosolized fecal material
Major respiratory diseases	Pneumonia, bronchitis, reactive airway disease	Pneumonia	Pneumonia

TABLE 2–5

Clinical Findings in Confirmed Human Psittacosis

SIGN OR SYMPTOM	% OF CASES
Fever	>95
Headache	>95
Chills	>95
Myalgias	>90
Sweats	50
Conjunctivitis or photophobia	50
Cough	50
Diarrhea or constipation	35
Leukopenia	25

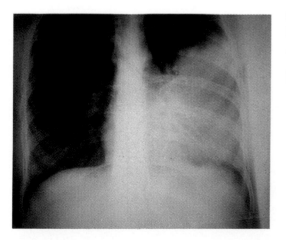

FIGURE 2–12

This patient had a large effusion complicating pneumonia due to *Mycoplasma pneumoniae.* This complication is not common.

FIGURE 2–13

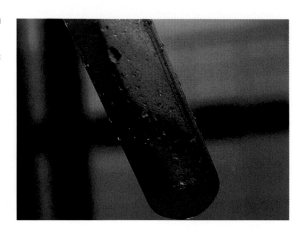

Bedside cold agglutinins are still used for a rapid diagnosis of *Mycoplasma* infections. Agglutination particles are seen in this tube, which had just been removed from the ice.

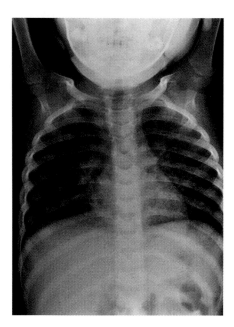

FIGURE 2–14

Measles pneumonia. This infant presented with pneumonia and the characteristic rash of measles.

ATYPICAL PNEUMONIA

TABLE 2–6

Conditions That Predispose to Aspiration

Altered consciousness
  Alcoholism, seizures, cerebrovascular accident, head trauma, general anesthesia, drug overdose
Dysphagia
  Esophageal stricture, neoplasm, or diverticula; tracheoesophageal fistula; incompetent cardiac sphincter
Gastroesophageal reflux
Neurologic disorder
  Multiple sclerosis, Parkinson disease, myasthenia gravis, pseudobulbar palsy
Mechanical disruption of the usual defense barriers
  Nasogastric tube, endotracheal intubation, tracheostomy, upper gastrointestinal endoscopy, bronchoscopy, protracted vomiting, gastric outlet obstruction, large-volume nasogastric tube feedings
Pharyngeal anesthesia
General debility
Recumbent position

TABLE 2–7

Differential Diagnosis of a Cavitary Lesion on Chest Radiograph

Necrotizing infections
Bacteria: anaerobes *Staphylococcus aureus,* enteric gram-negative bacteria, *Pseudomonas aeruginosa, Legionella* spp., *Haemophilus influenzae, Streptococcus pyogenes, Streptococcus pneumoniae (?), Rhodococcus, Actinomyces*
Mycobacteria: *Mycobacterium tuberculosis, Mycobacterium kansasii, Mycobacterium avium-intracellulare*
Bacteria-like: *Nocardia* spp.
Fungi: *Coccidioides immitis, Histoplasma capsulatum, Blastomyces hominis, Aspergillus* spp., *Mucor* spp.
Parasitic: *Entamoeba histolytica, Paragonimus westermani, Echinococcus*
Cavitary infarction
Bland infarction (with or without superimposed infection)
Septic embolism
S. aureus, anaerobes, others
Vasculitis
Wegener granulomatosis, periarteritis
Neoplasms
Bronchogenic carcinoma, metastatic carcinoma, lymphoma
Miscellaneous lesions
Cysts, blebs, bullae, or pneumatocele with or without fluid collections
Sequestration
Empyema with air-fluid level
Bronchiectasis

TABLE 2–8

Bacteriology of Lung Abscess

Total Cases	93
Aerobic bacteria only	10 (11%)
Anaerobic bacteria only	43 (46%)
Mixed aerobes-anaerobes	40 (43%)
Predominant Isolates	
Aerobes	
Staphylococcus aureus	13 (4)*
Escherichia coli	9
Klebsiella pneumoniae	7 (3)
Pseudomonas aeruginosa	7 (1)
Streptococcus pneumoniae	6 (1)
Anaerobes	
Peptostreptococcus spp.	40 (12)
Fusobacterium nucleatum	34 (5)
Prevotella melaninogenica	32 (1)
Bacteroides fragilis group	14

*Frequency of isolation; number in parentheses is frequency of isolation in pure culture.
Adapted from Bartlett JG: Anaerobic bacterial infections of the lung. Chest 91:901, 1987.

FIGURE 2–15

Lateral chest radiograph shows a lung abscess with an air fluid level. This patient experienced fevers and chest pain and produced foul smelling putrid sputum.

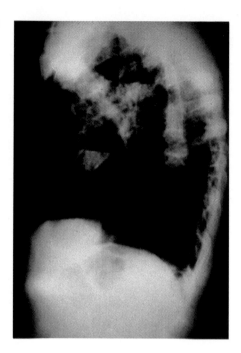

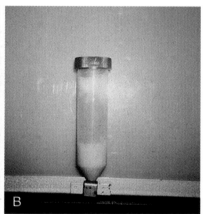

FIGURE 2–16

Needle aspiration of a lung abscess. Extended use of antibiotics is often sufficient to cure most lung abscesses. On occasion, surgical resection is required.

FIGURE 2–17

Empyema is a complication of *Staphylococcus aureus* pneumonia. This patient had an empyema requiring chest tube drainage.

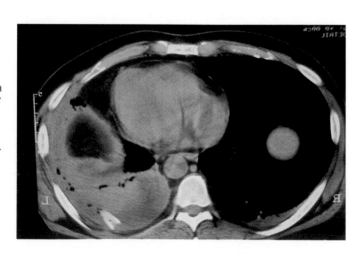

ASPIRATION AND COMPLICATIONS

TABLE 2–9

Comparison of Actinomycosis and Nocardiosis

PARAMETER	ACTINOMYCOSIS	NOCARDIOSIS
Agents	*Actinomyces israelii, Actinomyces naeslundii, Actinomyces odontolyticus, Actinomyces viscosus, Actinomyces meyeri, Propionibacterium propionicum*	*Nocardia asteroides*
Culture	Anaerobic (except *A. viscosus*)	Aerobic
Gram stain	Thin, branching, gram-positive bacilli	Thin, branching, gram-positive bacilli
Modified acid-fast stain	Negative	Positive
Source	Mouth, colon, genital tract	Soil
Host	Usually previously healthy young adult	Immunocompromised, especially reduced cell-mediated immunity
Pathophysiologic process	Endogenous infection starting in oval cavity, lung (aspiration), abdomen, or genital tract	Pneumonia presumably by inhalation; dissemination to extrapulmonary sites
Characteristic of infection	Indurated, draining sinuses, sulfur granules, penetration through tissue	No sulfur granules, penetration through tissue is unusual
Course	Indolent, chronic	Acute, subacute, or asymptomatic

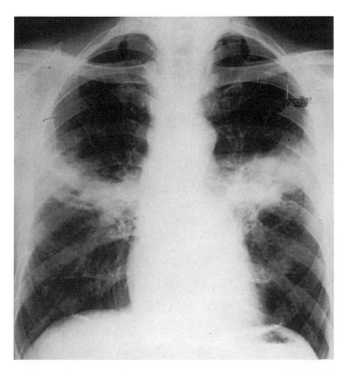

FIGURE 2–18

Nocardia pneumonia complicating corticosteroid treatment of polyarteritis.

FIGURE 2–19

Nocardia in sputum. (Gram stain.)

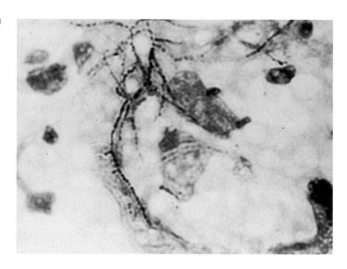

TABLE 2–10

Conditions Associated with *Nocardia*

Pulmonary alveolar proteinosis
Malignancy
Acquired immunodeficiency syndrome
Corticosteroid therapy
Cushing's syndrome
Organ transplantation
Chronic granulomatous disease of childhood
Congenital immunodeficiency diseases   ■

FIGURE 2–20

Nocardia growing in culture showing orange colonies after 7 days' growth.

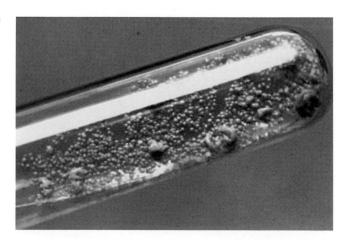

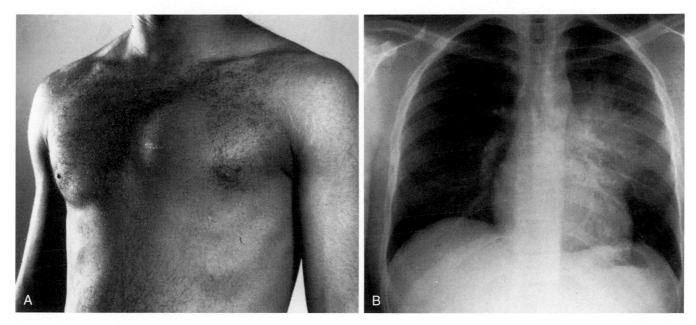

Thoracic actinomycosis. **A,** Initial presentation with a bulging mass lesion in the left chest wall with a central sinus tract. **B,** The associated pulmonary infiltrate shown on chest radiograph.

FIGURE 2–21

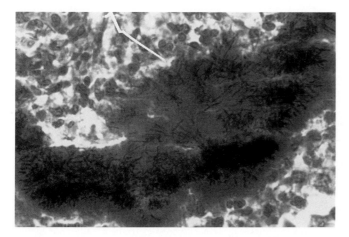

FIGURE 2–22

Sulfur granule or grain showing amorphous material with a rosette of filamentous, radiating gram-positive bacilli.

Nocardiosis and Actinomycosis

Infections of higher bacteria are often confused with one another; however, these organisms are quite different in their appearance and biology and in the diseases they cause.

TABLE 2–11

Fungi, Yeasts, and Higher Bacteria That Cause Pneumonia

MOSTLY IN NORMAL HOSTS	ABOUT EQUALLY IN NORMAL AND COMPROMISED PERSONS	MOSTLY IN COMPROMISED HOSTS
Histoplasma capsulatum	*Cryptococcus neoformans*	*Aspergillus* sp.
Blastomyces dermatitidis	*Nocardia asteroides*	Zygomycetes
Coccidioides immitis	*Sporothrix schenckii*	*Pseudallescheria boydii*
Actinomyces sp.	*Penicillium marneffei*	*Curvularia lunata*
	Geotrichum sp.	*Scopulariopsis* sp.
		Fusarium sp.
		Paecilomyces varioti
		Candida sp.
		Trichosporon sp.
		Candida (Torulopsis) glabrata

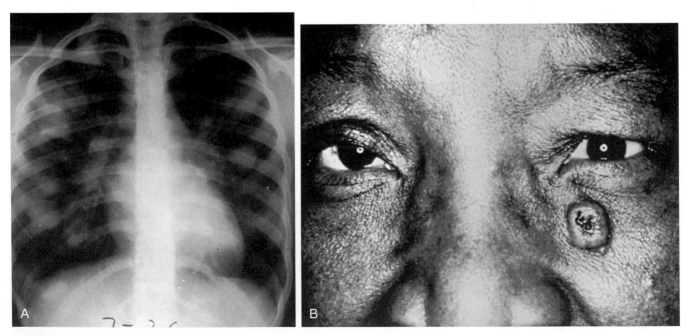

FIGURE 2–23   Cryptococcal nodular lung lesions **(A)** and ulcerating skin nodules **(B)** in a 72-year-old woman during steroid treatment for chronic lymphatic leukemia.

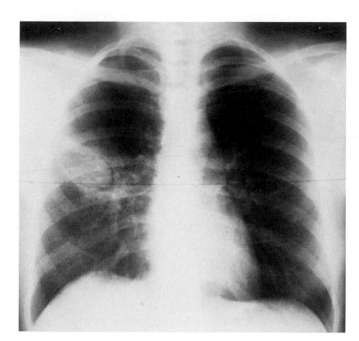

FIGURE 2–24

Aspergillus pneumonia presenting as an infarctlike lesion in a patient with subacute myelogenous leukemia after antileukemia therapy and multiple antibiotics for bacterial sepsis. (Courtesy of Dr. Donald Armstrong, Memorial Sloan-Kettering Cancer Center, New York, New York).

FIGURE 2–25

Huge aspergilloma within a lung cyst. (Courtesy of Dr. Baynard Tynes, University of Alabama School of Medicine, Birmingham, Alabama.)

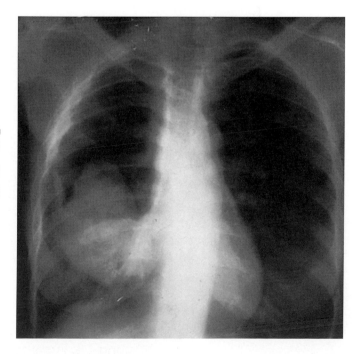

FIGURE 2–26

Aspergillus fumigatus. A posteroanterior chest radiograph from a 20-year-old woman marijuana smoker with *Aspergillus fumigatus* in sputum and recurrent wheezing and fever. Bilateral upper lobe infiltrates with prominence on right and cavitation are seen. Antibacterial and prednisone therapy given for allergic bronchopulmonary aspergillosis led to resolution.

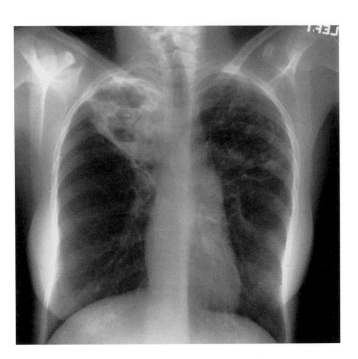

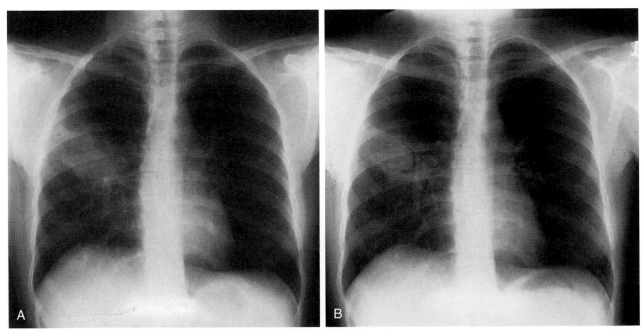

FIGURE 2–27

Posteroanterior chest radiographs from a 28-year-old woman with acute myelogenous leukemia and granulocytopenia show wedge-shaped right upper lobe infiltrate **(A)** and air-crescent sign around sequestrum **(B)**. Surgical resection was curative with remission of leukemia. (From Meyer RD, Young LS, Armstrong D, Yu B: Aspergillosis complicating neoplastic disease. Am J Med 54:6–15, 1973. With permission from Excerpta Medica Inc.)

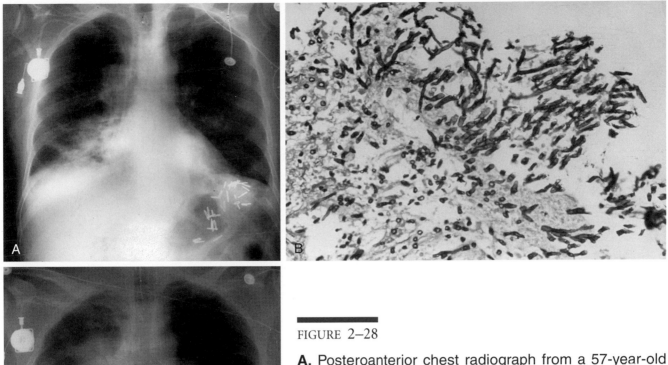

FIGURE 2–28

A, Posteroanterior chest radiograph from a 57-year-old man with granulocytopenia and lymphoma (undergoing methylprednisolone therapy) shows a hazy nodular right lower lobe and right upper lobe infiltrates that developed over 2 weeks. **B,** Histopathologic examination of a transbronchial biopsy specimen shows hyphae of aspergilli (cytologic preparation of bronchoalveolar lavage specimen also showed hyphae). **C,** Fatal progression of infiltrates followed despite amphotericin B therapy.

FIGURE 2–29

Outcome of infection. (Based on data from Smith CE, Beard RR, Whiting EG, Rosenberger HG: Varieties of coccidioidal infection in relation to the epidemiology and control of disease. Am J Public Health 36:1394, 1946.)

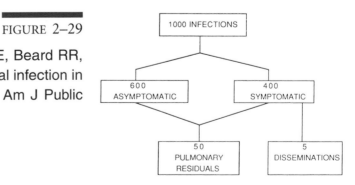

FIGURE 2–30

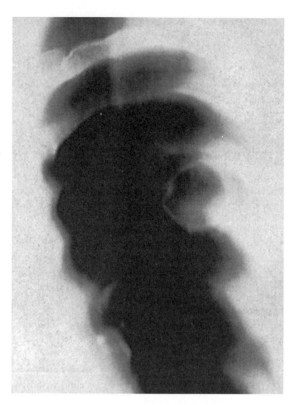

Thin-walled pulmonary cavity caused by *Coccidioides immitis*. (Courtesy of Dr. David Stevens, Santa Clara Valley Medical Center, San Jose, California.)

FIGURE 2–31

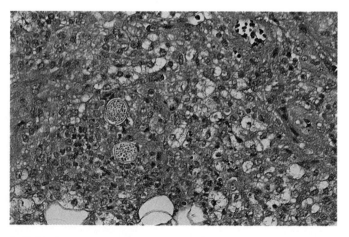

Histology of this lung specimen reveals many large endosporulating spherules. No granulomas are seen.

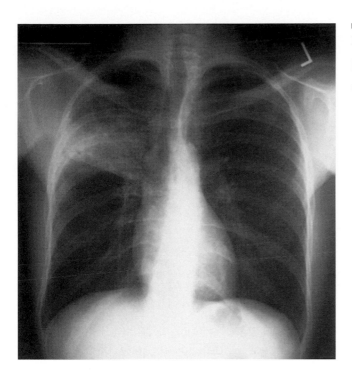

FIGURE 2–32

Pulmonary blastomycosis. Airspace disease is apparent in the right upper lobe.

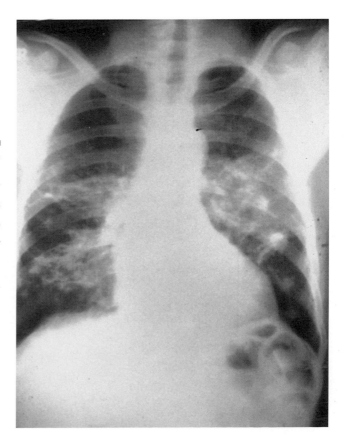

FIGURE 2–33

Pulmonary paracoccidioidomycosis. The chest radiograph reveals bilateral interstitial and alveolar infiltrates in the middle and lower lobes. The upper lobes are spared. (Courtesy of Angela Restrepo, PhD, Mycology Unit, Corporacìon des Investigaciones Biológicas, Medellín, Colombia.)

FIGURE 2–34

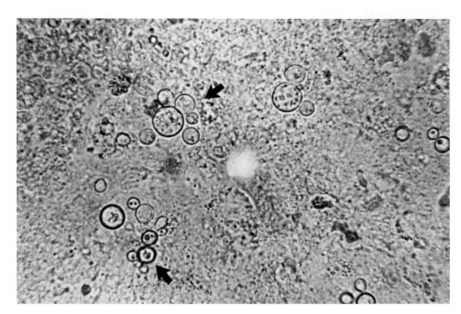

Paracoccidioides brasiliensis yeasts in potassium hydroxide–treated sputum sample. Arrows point to the pilot wheel appearance of the fungus. (Courtesy of Angela Restrepo, PhD, Mycology Unit, Corporacìon des Investigaciones Biológicas, Medellín, Colombia.)

FIGURE 2–35

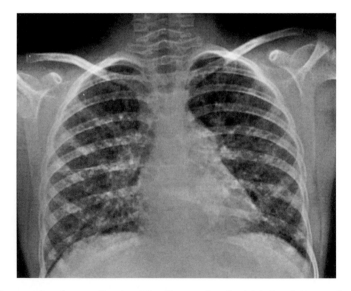

Chest radiograph of a patient with disseminated histoplasmosis shows diffuse interstitial alveolar infiltrates.

3

ENDOVASCULAR INFECTIONS

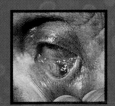
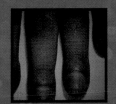
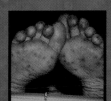

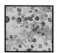 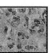 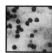

Cutaneous signs of bacteremia may be hard to discern. Discovery of splinter hemorrhages, Roth spots, or conjunctival hemorrhages will help establish an early diagnosis of endocarditis. Clinicians must be aware of the subtle findings of endovascular infections.

VASCULAR GRAFT INFECTIONS

TABLE 3–1

Bacteriology of Graft Infection

| | TYPES OF BACTERIA IN CULTURE (%) | | | | | | |
ORGANISM	Bandyk et al (1984) (n = 30)	Bunt (1983) (n = 205)	Calligaro et al (1990) (n = 30)	Cherry et al (1992) (n = 39)	Liekweg and Greenfield (1977) (n = 22)	Quinones-Baldrich et al (1991) (n = 45)	Szilagyi et al (1972) (n = 48)
Staphylococcus (coagulase-positive)	8	43	24	31	41	13	33
Staphylococcus (coagulase-negative)	42	—	24	10	—	21	15
Streptococcus (nonhemolytic)	6	—	51	18	—	5	5
Escherichia coli	11	17	10	(28% gram-negative)	9	18	23
Proteus	—	8	20		1	5	6
Pseudomonas	3	10	33	8	14	21	2
Mixed				20		39	
Negative culture				10		21	∎

TABLE 3–2

Clinical Diagnosis of Graft Infections (Average from Literature)

TYPE OF INFECTION	%
General	
Localized cellulitis or abscess	50
Fever	37
Systemic infection	25
Leukocytosis	26
Draining sinus	20
False aneurysm	16
Anastomotic bleeding	12
Graft occlusion	8
Septic emboli	6
Aortic Level	
Herald bleeding	76
Acute gastrointestinal bleeding	56
Chronic gastrointestinal bleeding	40

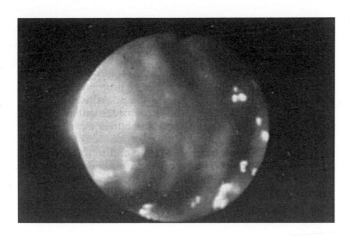

FIGURE 3–1

Endoscopic view of an aortoenteric fistula. Whitish, highly reflective material at 9 o'clock position represents graft fabric; mucosa with hemorrhage is seen to fill the remainder of the circle.

FIGURE 3–2

Obvious extrusion of graft through inguinal wound in a patient with a draining sinus and graft infection. This patient had had an aortofemoral bypass graft several years earlier and was referred for management of this infection.

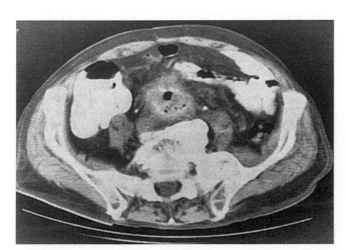

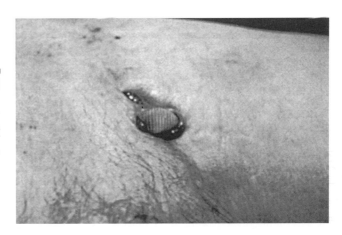

FIGURE 3–3

Computed tomographic scan of a patient with a graft infection. Blurring of the usual tissue planes in the retroperitoneum, as well as air, is observed around the shaft of the aortic graft.

FIGURE 3–4

Computed tomographic scan of a false aneurysm in a patient with an aortoenteric fistula. The aortic anastomotic aneurysm was inferential evidence of a suspected aortoenteric fistula. This view above the graft anastomosis reveals the false aneurysm and overlying bowel.

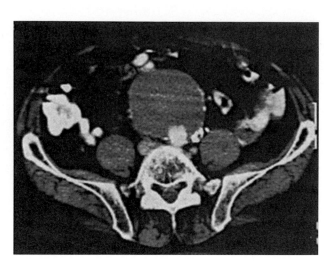

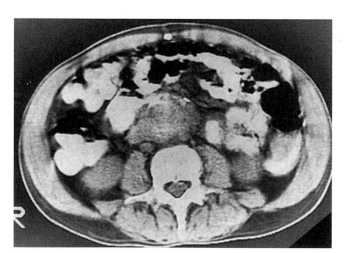

FIGURE 3–5

Computed tomographic scan of an aortoenteric fistula with oral contrast medium from the duodenum delineating the aortic graft (11 o'clock position of the graft).

FIGURE 3–6

Upper gastrointestinal tract series in a patient with an aortoenteric fistula. The drawing on the right illustrates the barium study on the left. The ulcer appeared in the fourth portion of the duodenum overlying the aortic anastomosis.

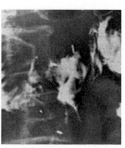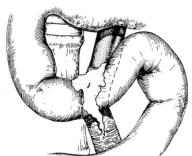

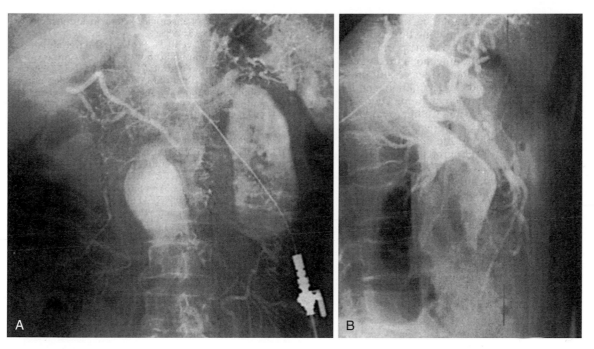

FIGURE 3–7

Anteroposterior **(A)** and lateral **(B)** arteriograms of a patient with an aortic false aneurysm and gastrointestinal bleeding. Subsequent exploration revealed an aortoenteric fistula, which was treated by graft excision and extraanatomic bypass by axillofemoral bypass.

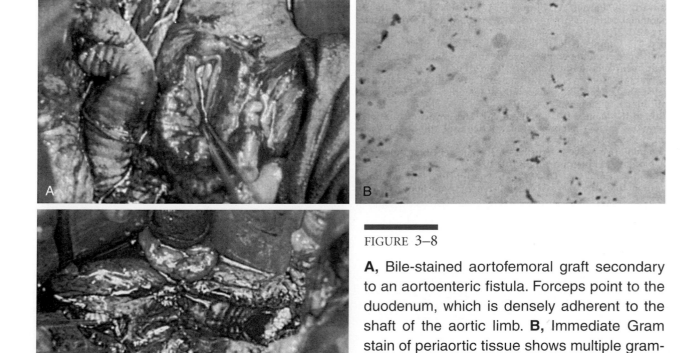

FIGURE 3–8

A, Bile-stained aortofemoral graft secondary to an aortoenteric fistula. Forceps point to the duodenum, which is densely adherent to the shaft of the aortic limb. **B,** Immediate Gram stain of periaortic tissue shows multiple gram-positive organisms. **C,** Completed aortic stump closure and fistula. Forceps point to open bowel, which subsequently was closed.

ENDOCARDITIS

TABLE 3–3

Microbiology of Prosthetic Valve Endocarditis, 1975 to 1989

ORGANISM	<2 Months N = 73	2–12 Months N = 38	>12 Months N = 94
Coagulase-negative staphylococci	28 (38)	19 (50)	14 (15)
Staphylococcus aureus	10 (14)	4 (11)	12 (13)
Gram-negative bacilli	8 (11)	2 (5)	1 (1)
Streptococci	0	1 (3)	31 (33)
Enterococci	5 (7)	2 (5)	10 (11)
Diphtheroids	9 (12)	1 (3)	2 (2)
Fastidious gram-negative coccobacilli	0	1 (3)	11 (12)
Fungi	7 (10)	2 (5)	3 (3)
Miscellaneous	3 (4)	2 (5)	1 (1)
Culture-negative	3 (4)	4 (11)	9 (10)

(NO. OF CASES (%) AT TIME OF ONSET AFTER CARDIAC SURGERY)

Adapted from Karchmer AW: Infective endocarditis. *In* Braunwald E (ed): Heart Disease, ed 5. Philadelphia, WB Saunders, 1997, pp 1077–1104.

TABLE 3–4

Frequency of Microbial Pathogens in Infective Endocarditis

ORGANISMS	NATIVE VALVE (%) Nonaddicts	Addicts	PROSTHETIC VALVE (%) Early (<2 mo)	Late (>2 mo)
Streptococci	50–70	20	5–10	25–30
Enterococci	10	8	<1	5–10
Staphylococci	25	60	45–50	30–40
S. aureus	23	59	15–20	10–12
S. epidermidis	2	1	25–30	23–28
Gram-negative bacilli	<1	10	20	10–12
Fungi	<1	5	10–12	5–8
Diphtheroids	<1	2	5–10	4–5
Miscellaneous organisms	5–10	1–5	1–5	1–5
Multiple organisms	<1	5	8	8
Culture-negative results	5–10	10–20	5–10	5–10

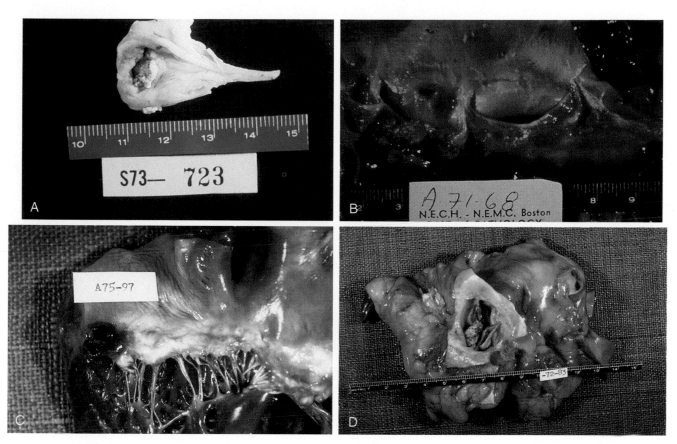

Gross specimens of cardiac vegetations. Note the irregular contour of the valve surfaces. **A,** The vegetation on the aortic valve is clearly shown. This patient has subacute bacterial endocarditis. **B,** Multiple vegetations are seen on this aortic valve cusp. **C,** This mitral valve was infected with *Staphylococcus aureus.* **D,** Aortic valve of a patient with subacute bacterial endocarditis due to *Haemophilus aphrophilus.* Note the large size of the vegetation, which is typical of this organism.

FIGURE 3–9

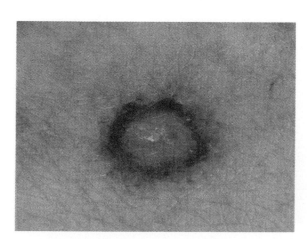

FIGURE 3–10

Skin lesion of a patient with acute bacterial endocarditis due to group G streptococci. Lesions of this size are rare. When present, they are usually painless.

FIGURE 3–11

Lower extremity petechial lesions in a patient with subacute bacterial endocarditis. Petechiae are present in as many as 40% of patients with endocarditis.

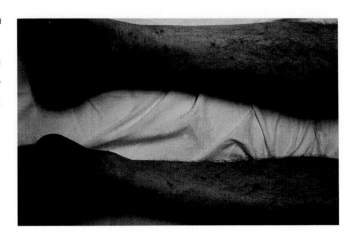

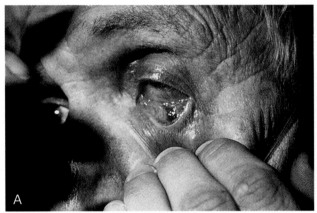
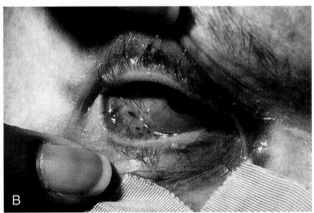

FIGURE 3–12

Conjunctival petechiae or hemorrhages are highly predictive of endocarditis. They must be carefully sought in suspected cases. (Courtesy of Dr. Mark Drapkin, Newton Wellesley Hospital, Newton, Massachusetts.)

FIGURE 3–13

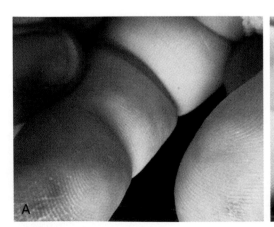
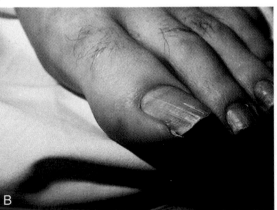

Osler nodes. These painful lesions on the extremities are found in no more than 25% of patients with endocarditis. They usually are found on a distal extremity.

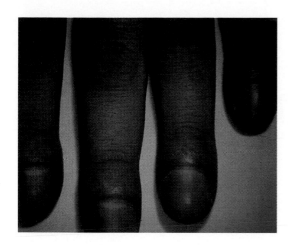

FIGURE 3–14

Clubbing. Signs of clubbing are seen in approximately 50% of patients with subacute bacterial endocarditis. Clubbing rapidly resolves after appropriate treatment.

FIGURE 3–15

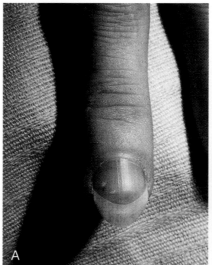

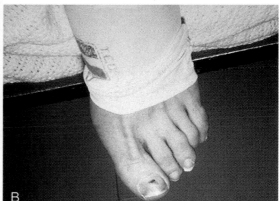

Splinter hemorrhages. A minority of patients with endocarditis have splinter hemorrhages, which often are difficult to find.

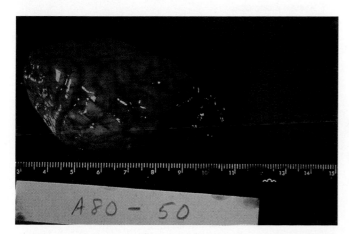

FIGURE 3–16

Rupture of a mycotic aneurysm is the most feared complication of endocarditis. These small, peripheral aneurysms occur in less than 10% of cases, but their rupture has devastating consequences.

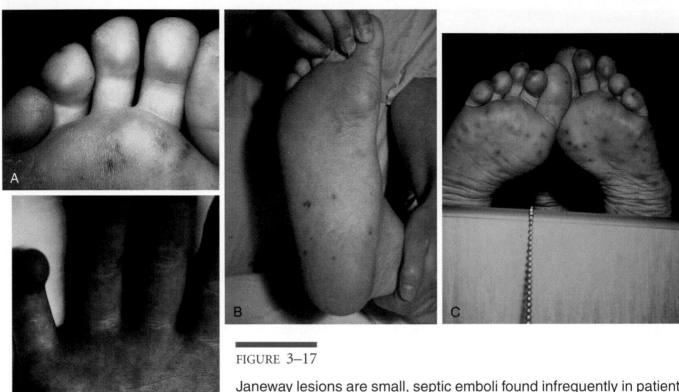

FIGURE 3–17

Janeway lesions are small, septic emboli found infrequently in patients with endocarditis. They are painless and are found on the palms or soles.

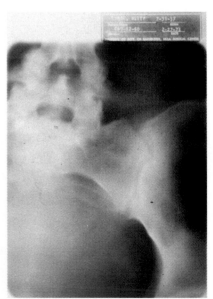

FIGURE 3–18

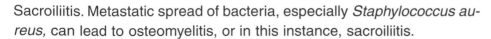

Sacroiliitis. Metastatic spread of bacteria, especially *Staphylococcus aureus,* can lead to osteomyelitis, or in this instance, sacroiliitis.

4

GASTROINTESTINAL AND ABDOMINAL INFECTIONS

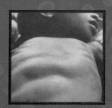 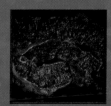 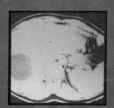

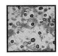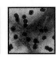

DISEASE OF THE INTESTINES

TABLE 4–1

Clinical Features of Acute Diarrhea

CLINICAL OBSERVATION	ANATOMIC CONSIDERATION	PATHOGENS TO CONSIDER
Passage of few, voluminous stools	Diarrhea of small bowel origin	*Vibrio cholerae,* enterotoxigenic *Escherichia coli, Shigella* strains early in the infection, *Giardia*
Passage of many small-volume stools	Diarrhea of large bowel origin	*Shigella, Salmonella, Campylobacter, Entamoeba histolytica*
Tenesmus, fecal urgency, dysentery	Colitis	*Shigella, Salmonella, Campylobacter, E. histolytica*
Vomiting as the predominant symptom	Gastroenteritis	Viral agents (rotavirus, Norwalk virus) or intoxication *(Staphylococcus aureus, Bacillus cereus)*
Fever as the predominant finding	Mucosal invasion	*Shigella, Salmonella, Campylobacter,* viral agents (rotavirus, Norwalk virus) ■

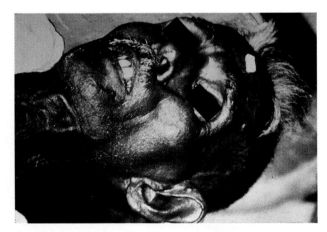

FIGURE 4–1

Cholera-dehydrated facies. Cholera chiefly affects the old and the young in developing countries. Dehydration is rapid.

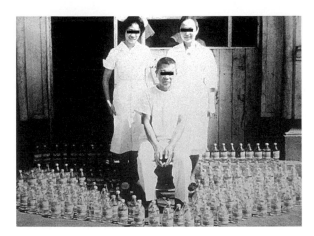

FIGURE 4–2

Amount of intravenous fluid needed to resuscitate one survivor of cholera. Oral rehydration is the standard therapy for most cases today.

TABLE 4–2

Clinical Presentations and Likely Agents of Acute Diarrheal Disease

CLINICAL TYPE	PATIENTS (APPROXIMATE %)	LIKELY AGENT* Industrialized Countries	Developing Countries
Simple diarrhea	90	Rotavirus, other viruses, *Salmonella, Campylobacter jejuni*	Rotavirus, ETEC, *C. jejuni*
Dysentery	5–10	*Shigella, C. jejuni*, EIEC, *Yersinia*	*Shigella, C. jejuni, Entamoeba histolytica*, EIEC
Persistent diarrhea (>14 d)	3–4	*Giardia, Salmonella, Yersinia*	EPEC, *Giardia*, EAggEC
Severe purging of rice-water stools	1†	Rotavirus, *Salmonella*	*Vibrio cholerae*, ETEC
Hemorrhagic colitis	<1	EHEC	EHEC, *Shigella dysenteriae* type 1
Repeated vomiting without diarrhea	1–2		
Acute	1	Norwalk virus, other viruses	Viruses, *Giardia*
Persistent	<0.5	*Giardia*	*Giardia, Strongyloides*

*ETEC, Enterotoxigenic *E. coli;* EIEC, enteroinvasive *E. coli;* EPEC, enteropathogenic *E. coli;* EHEC, enterohemorrhagic *E. coli;* EAggEC, enteroaggregative *E. coli.*
†More common in cholera endemic areas.

FIGURE 4–3

Salmonella isolation rates in the United States, by age and sex of patient and year, 1970 and 1986. (From Harrett-Bean NT, Pavia AT, Tauxe RV: *Salmonella* isolates from humans in the United States, 1984–1986. MMWR CDC Surveill Summ 2:25–31, 1988.)

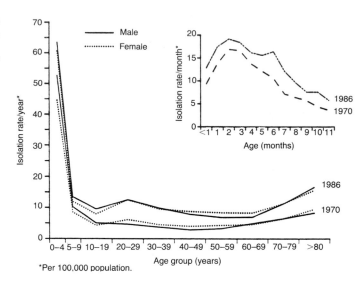

*Per 100,000 population.

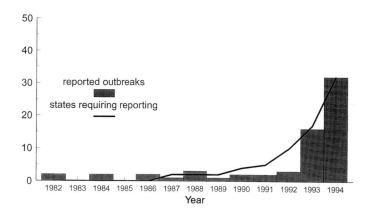

FIGURE 4–4

Number of outbreaks of *E. coli* O157:H7 infection reported to the Centers of Disease Control and Prevention and the number of states requiring reporting of *E. coli* O157:H7 infections, 1982 to 1994.

FIGURE 4–5

Encephalopathic manifestations of *Shigella flexneri* infection. Posturing, staring, and unresponsiveness can be appreciated in this Bangladeshi child. (Courtesy of Dr. Michael L. Bennish, New England Medical Center, Boston, Massachusetts.)

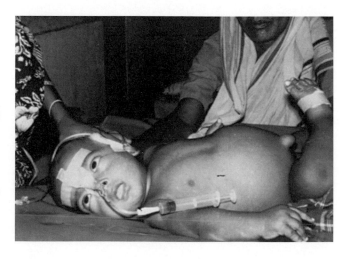

TABLE 4–3

Clinical Features Associated with *Campylobacter* and Related Species Implicated as Causes of Human Illness

SPECIES	COMMONLY ENCOUNTERED CLINICAL FEATURES	LESS COMMONLY ENCOUNTERED CLINICAL FEATURES
C. jejuni	Fever, diarrhea, abdominal pain	Bacteremia
C. coli	Fever, diarrhea, abdominal pain	Bacteremia
C. fetus	Bacteremia, sepsis, meningitis, vascular infections	Diarrhea, relapsing fevers
C. upsaliensis	Watery diarrhea, low-grade fever, abdominal pain	Bacteremia, abscesses
C. lari	Gastroenteritis, abdominal pain, diarrhea	Colitis, appendicitis
C. hyointestinalis	Watery or bloody diarrhea, vomiting, abdominal pain	Bacteremia
Helicobacter fennelliae	Chronic, mild diarrhea; abdominal cramps; proctitis	Bacteremia in persons infected with human immunodeficiency virus and in children
Helicobacter cinaedi	Chronic, mild diarrhea; abdominal cramps; proctitis	Bacteremia in persons infected with human immunodeficiency virus and in children
C. jejuni subsp. *doylei*	Gastroenteritis	Chronic gastritis, bacteremia in children
Arcobacter cryaerophilus	Gastroenteritis	Bacteremia
Arcobacter butzleri	Fever, diarrhea, abdominal pain, nausea	Bacteremia, appendicitis
C. sputorum	Lung, perianal, groin, axillary abscesses	
Hydrogen-requiring *Campylobacter* species*	Periodontitis	Diarrhea, osteomyelitis, bacteremia in children

*Includes *C. rectus, C. curvus,* and *C. concisus.*

TABLE 4–4

Spectrum of *Yersinia enterocolitica* Infections

Gastrointestinal Infections
Enterocolitis, especially in young children; concomitant bacteremia may also be present
Pseudoappendicitis syndrome (children older than 5 y; adults)
   Acute mesenteric lymphadenitis
   Terminal ileitis

Septicemia
Especially in immunosuppressed individuals and those with iron overload or being treated with desferrioxamine
Transfusion related

Metastatic Infections after Septicemia
Focal abscesses: liver, kidney, spleen, lung
Cutaneous manifestations: cellulitis, pyomyositis, pustules and bullous lesions
Pneumonia, cavitary pneumonia
Meningitis
Panophthalmitis
Endocarditis, infected mycotic aneurysm
Osteomyelitis

Postinfection Sequelae Associated with Human Leukocyte Antigen B27
Arthritis
Myocarditis
Glomerulonephritis
Erthema nodosum

Pharyngitis

FIGURE 4–6

Toxic megacolon due to shigellosis in a Bangladeshi infant. The dilated bowel is easily seen. (From Keusch GT, Formal SB, Bennish ML: Shigellosis. *In* Warren KS, Mahmoud AAF [eds]: Tropical and Geographical Medicine, Vol 2. New York, McGraw-Hill, 1990, pp 762–776.)

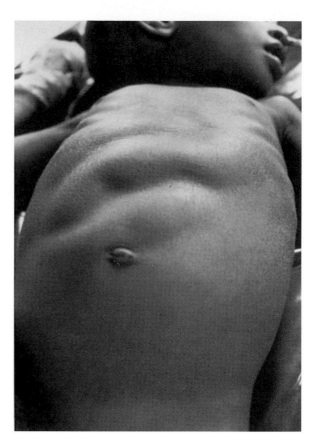

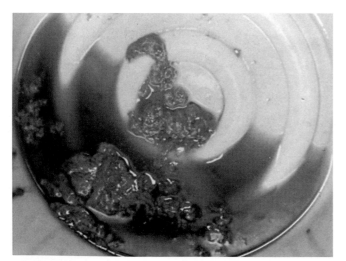

FIGURE 4–7

A characteristic stool of shigellosis, with mucoid stool mixed with a small amount of bloody fluid. The typical dysenteric stool, consisting of a small amount of grossly bloody mucus, is actually uncommon. (From Keusch GT, Formal SB, Bennish ML: Shigellosis. *In* Warren KS, Mahmoud AAF [eds]: Tropical and Geographical Medicine, Vol 2. New York, McGraw-Hill, 1990, pp 762–776.)

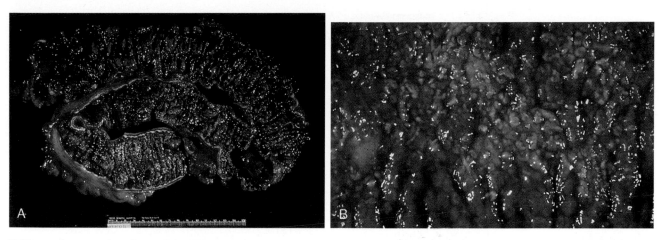

Diffuse hemorrhagic colitis. This resected specimen of colon shows a diffuse hemorrhagic colitis. The close-up reveals the diffuse mucosal irregularity and pseudomembrane formation.

FIGURE 4–8

FIGURE 4–9

This computed tomographic scan of abdomen shows colitis due to *Clostridium difficile* with thickened colonic mucosa.

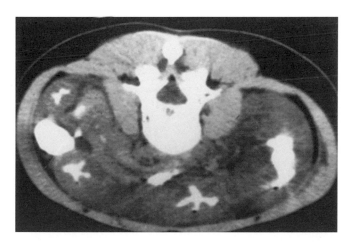

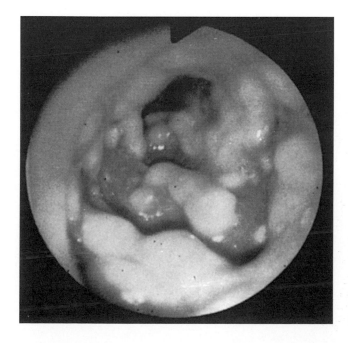

FIGURE 4–10

Pseudomembranous plaques seen with colonoscopy in a patient with *C. difficile*–associated pseudomembranous colitis.

FIGURE 4–11

Morphologic types of *Giardia.* Diagrammatic representation of light microscopic appearances of *G. agilis, G. muris,* and *G. intestinalis.* N, Nucleus; MB, median body; F, flagellum.

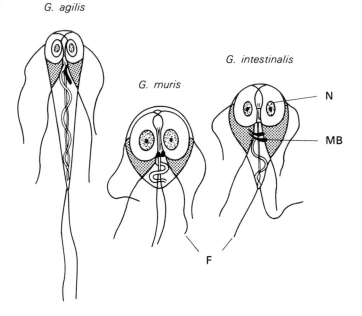

FIGURE 4–12

Barium follow-through examination in a man with chronic giardiasis and hypogammaglobulinemia, showing diffuse lymphoid nodular hyperplasia throughout the small intestine.

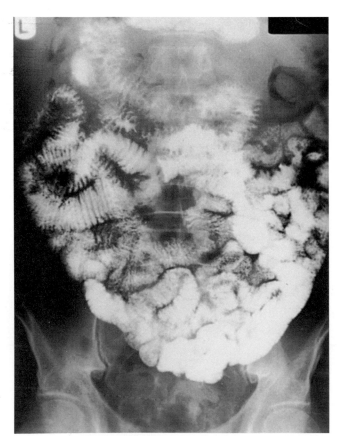

TABLE 4–5

Microbial Pathogens in Traveler's Diarrhea

	FREQUENCY	
PATHOGEN	Average (%)	Range (%)
Enterotoxigenic *Escherichia coli*	40–60	0–72
Enteroadherent *E. coli*	15	—
Invasive *E. coli*	<5	0–5
Shigella	10	0–30
Salmonella	<5	0–15
Campylobacter	<5	0–15
Vibrio	<5	0–30
Aeromonas	<5	0–30
Rotavirus	5	0–36
Giardia lamblia	<5	0–6
Entamoeba histolytica	<5	0–6
Cryptosporidium	<5	—
No pathogen identified	40	22–83 ■

TABLE 4–6

Pathogens of 900 Intraabdominal Infections Isolated in Six Independent Studies

	ISOLATES	
PATHOGEN	Number	%
Aerobes		
Escherichia coli	462	38
Klebsiella species	129	10
Enterobacter species	56	5
Proteus species	141	11
Pseudomonas aeruginosa	63	5
Staphylococcus aureus	46	4
Enterococcus faecalis	150	12
Other streptococci	107	9
Other aerobes	75	6
Total	1229	48
Anaerobes		
Bacteroides fragilis	329	24
Other *Bacteroides* species	318	24
Fusobacteria	61	5
Veillonella	22	2
Peptococci	71	5
Peptostreptococci	113	8
Clostridia	205	15
Propionibacteria	41	3
Other	189	14
Total	1349	52
Grand total	2578	■

Data from Wittmann DH: Treatment of Peritonitis: Antibiotic Concentration Dynamics at the Site of Infection as Criterion of Antimicrobial Chemotherapy. Habilitation. Hamburg, Medizinische Fakultät der Universität, 1985. Thesis.

FIGURE 4–13

In this patient with peritonitis, preoperative chest radiograph demonstrates free air under both hemidiaphragms.

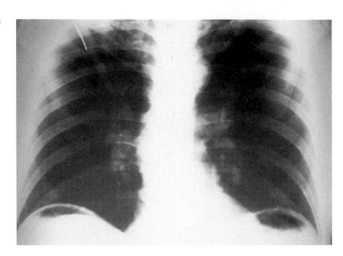

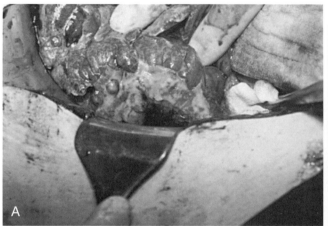

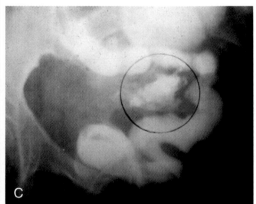

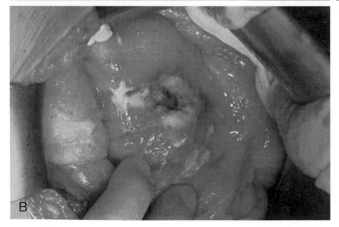

FIGURE 4–14

Peritonitis caused by perforated diverticulum. **A,** Peritonitis with fibrinous exudate and diverticula of the sigmoid colon. **B,** Inflammation of the peritoneum caused by a perforated diverticulum of the sigmoid colon. **C,** Radiograph revealing extravasated diatrizoate (Gastrografin) from a perforated diverticulum.

DISEASES OF THE LIVER, SPLEEN, AND PANCREAS

TABLE 4–7

Microorganisms Found in 45 Pancreatic Infections*

ORGANISM	NO. OF SPECIMENS
Escherichia	22
Enterococcus	17
Staphylococcus	16
Klebsiella	6
Proteus	4
Candida albicans	3
Pseudomonas	3
Streptococcus	2
Torulopsis glabrata	1
Haemophilus parainfluenzae	1
Diphtheroids	1
Serratia marcescens	1
Negative culture (positive Gram stain for organisms on smear)	5

*More than one organism was propagated from 20 specimens.

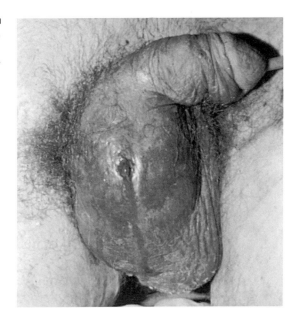

FIGURE 4–15

Retroperitoneal extension of a pancreatic abscess necessitating out through the scrotum.

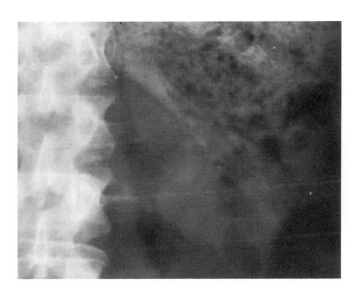

FIGURE 4–16

Abdominal radiograph shows the classic soap bubble sign of a pancreatic abscess.

FIGURE 4–22

Acute cholecystitis with an obstructing stone at the neck of the gallbladder, which is thick walled and edematous, with serosal inflammation.

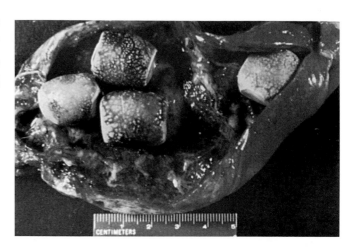

TABLE 4–9

Microbiology of Splenic Abscess

BACTERIAL FINDINGS	%*
Aerobic Bacteria	59.4
Streptococcus	16.0
Staphylococcus	14.7
Salmonella	7.3
Other Gram-Negative Bacteria	21.4
Escherichia coli	36.0
Proteus	20.0
Shigella	18.0
Klebsiella	2.0
Unspecified coliforms	6.0
Pseudomonas	2.0
Anaerobes	12.1
Mixed organisms	32.0
Bacteroides	25.0
Propionibacterium	21.0
Clostridium	14.0
Streptococcus	11.0
Fusobacterium	4.0
Fungi	2.4
Sterile Cultures	26.6

*N = 230.

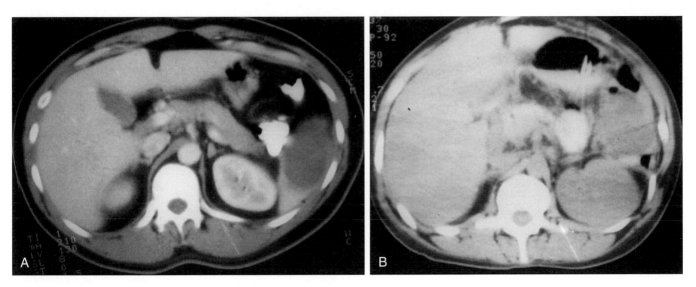

A, Unilocular hypodense splenic abscess secondary to endocarditis. The infecting organism was *Staphylococcus.* The patient was treated successfully with a splenectomy. **B,** A hypodense spleen with an air bubble seen on a computed tomographic scan. The contiguous colonic and pancreatic process mandated a splenectomy. Multiple enteric organisms were cultured.

FIGURE 4–23

TABLE 4–10

Bacteriology of Liver Abscess: 25 Cases Involving Anaerobic Bacteria

BACTERIA	NUMBER OF LIVER ISOLATES	NUMBER OF BLOOD ISOLATES
Anaerobes	30	14
Peptostreptococci	6	2
Microaerophilic streptococci	7	7
Fusobacteria	5	1
Bacteroides fragilis	5	2
Other *Bacteroides* sp.	5	2
Aerobes	7	6
Streptococci	4	3
Escherichia coli	2	2
Proteus	1	0

From Sabbaj J, Sutter VL, Finegold SM: Anaerobic pyogenic liver abscess. Ann Intern Med 77:629, 1972.

FIGURE 4–24

Magnetic resonance image shows a large hepatic abscess.

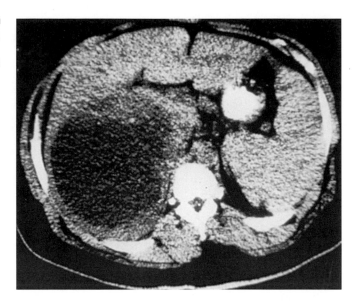

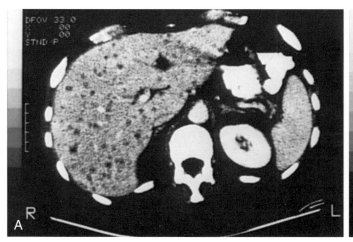

FIGURE 4–25

Computed tomographic scan of the liver of a patient with hepatic candidiasis before and after recovery from neutropenia. **A,** At time of diagnosis. **B,** One month later, after treatment with intravenous amphotericin B.

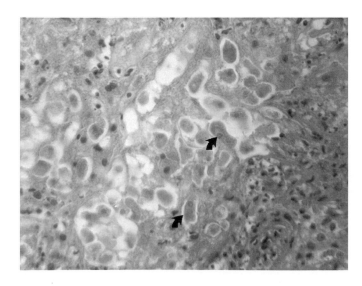

FIGURE 4–26

Pathology of amebic liver abscess. The section shows necrotic liver with trophozoites *(arrows)* at the edge of the abscess. The clear halo around the trophozoite is a common fixation artifact. (H&E, × 100.)

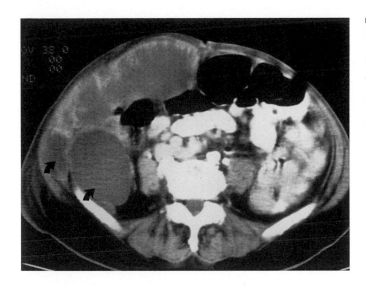

FIGURE 4–27

Computed tomographic scan shows localized rupture of an amebic liver abscess *(arrows).* (Courtesy of Department of Radiology, University of California at San Diego Medical Center, San Diego, California.)

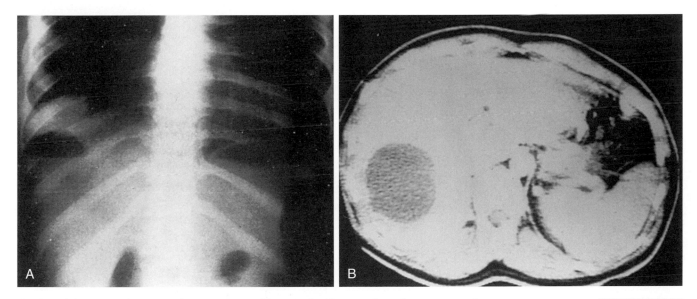

A, Amebic liver abscess demonstrated by aspiration and replacement of aspirated material with air. Note the location in the right lobe of the liver. **B,** Amebic liver abscess documented by computed tomography. (Courtesy of Dr. J. J. Marr, Immunologic Pharmaceutical Corp., Waltham, Massachusetts.)

FIGURE 4–28

FIGURE 4–29

Swelling over the liver may be an important sign of a large amebic liver abscess. It may present months, or even years, after a person has left an area endemic for the disease.

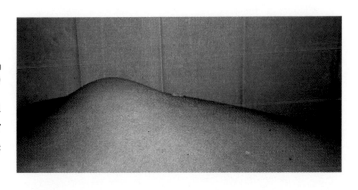

FIGURE 4–30

Aspiration of fluid from an amebic liver abscess. The fluid contains few organisms. In most instances, serology will establish the diagnosis, and aspiration will not be necessary.

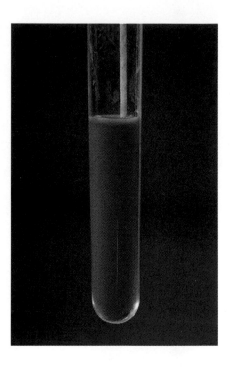

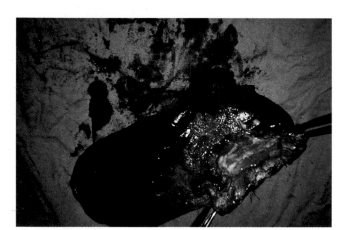

FIGURE 4–31

Surgical removal of an amebic liver abscess should be considered only if there is no response to therapy or if there is fear that the abscess will rupture into the pericardium from the left lobe of the liver. Great care must be taken to avoid spillage of contaminated fluid into the peritoneum.

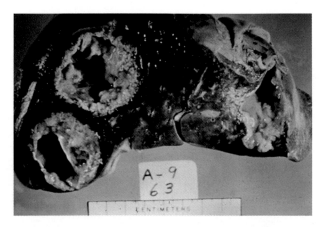

FIGURE 4–32

Amebic thick-walled abscess. This pathologic specimen reveals multiple liver abscesses due to *Entamoeba histolytica*.

5

SEXUALLY
TRANSMITTED
DISEASES

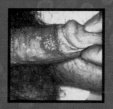 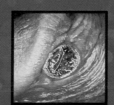 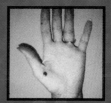

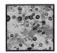 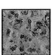

When confronted with a patient with a genital lesion it is important to determine the nature of the lesion and whether it may have been transmitted sexually. Recognition and treatment are often necessary on the first visit before any results are available. Partner notification may be required in some instances.

TABLE 5–1

Sexually Transmitted Pathogens, Copathogens, and Clinical Syndromes*

SYNDROME	PRIMARY PATHOGENS	SECONDARY PATHOGENS AND COPATHOGENS
Acquired immunodeficiency syndrome and related disorders	HIV (types 1 and 2)	Numerous opportunistic pathogens
Acute pelvic inflammatory disease and its primary complications, female infertility, ectopic pregnancy, chronic pelvic pain	*Neisseria gonorrhoeae, Chlamydia trachomatis*	*Mycoplasma hominis, Prevotella* sp., *Peptococcus* sp., *Bacteroides* sp., coliform bacteria, other vaginal flora
Neonatal or perinatal complications (premature delivery, chorioamnionitis, TORCHES syndrome, pneumonia, conjunctivitis, cognitive impairment, immunodeficiency)	*N. gonorrhoeae, C. trachomatis,* CMV, HSV (types 1 and 2), *Treponema pallidum,* group B streptococcus, HIV	*Ureaplasma urealyticum, M. hominis,* vaginal anaerobes
Neoplasia (squamous cell cancer of cervix, anus, vulva, penis; Kaposi's sarcoma; lymphoma; hepatocellular carcinoma)	Human papillomavirus (types 16, 18, 34, 45, others), HIV, hepatitis B virus, Kaposi's sarcoma virus	
Lower genital tract infections in women		
Mucopurulent cervicitis and urethritis	*C. trachomatis, N. gonorrhoeae,* HSV	*Trichomonas vaginalis*
Vaginitis, vulvovaginitis	*Trichomonas vaginalis, Candida* sp.	Anaerobic vaginal flora, other yeasts
Bacterial vaginosis	Primary pathogen(s) unknown	*Gardnerella vaginalis, M. hominis, Mobiluncus* sp., anaerobic vaginal flora
Anogenital warts	Human papillomaviruses (especially types 6 and 11)	
Viral hepatitis	Hepatitis viruses (A, B, C, D)	
Male urethritis	*N. gonorrhoeae, C. trachomatis, U. urealyticum* (?), *Mycoplasma genitalium* (?)	*T. vaginalis,* HSV-1 and HSV-2
Genital ulcer–lymphadenopathy syndromes	*T. pallidum,* HSV-1, HSV-2, *Haemophilus ducreyi, C. trachomatis* (LGV strains), *Calymmatobacterium granulomatis*	Pyogenic bacteria, *Candida* sp., other fungi
Arthritis	*N. gonorrhoeae, C. trachomatis,* hepatitis B virus, HIV (?)	*U. urealyticum, M. hominis*
Epididymitis	*C. trachomatis, N. gonorrhoeae*	Genitourinary pathogens
Tertiary syphilis	*T. pallidum*	
Proctitis, proctocolitis	Same as for urethritis, cervicitis	
Enteric infections, enterocolitis	*Shigella* sp., *Giardia lamblia, Entamoeba histolytica, Campylobacter* sp., HIV (?)	
Mononucleosis	CMV, human herpesvirus type 6 (?), Epstein-Barr virus, HIV (?)	
Ectoparasite infestation	*Sarcoptes scabiei* (scabies mite), *Phthirus pubis* (crab louse)	Pyogenic bacteria
Molluscum contagiosum	Molluscum contagiosum virus	

*Listed in approximate order of importance to human health. TORCHES, Toxoplasmosis, rubella, cytomegalovirus, herpes, syphilis; HIV, human immunodeficiency virus; CMV, cytomegalovirus; HSV, herpes simplex virus; LGV, lymphogranuloma venereum.

HERPES SIMPLEX

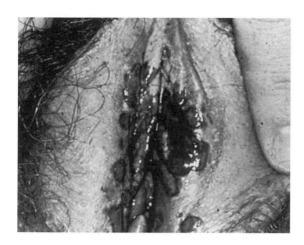

FIGURE 5–1

Primary genital herpes in the female patient. This young woman with primary herpetic vulvovaginitis has shallow, exquisitely tender ulcers on the inner surface of the labia majora, the labia minora, and the vaginal mucosa. The ulcers are covered with a yellowish gray exudate and surrounded by a narrow zone of erythema. Further examination also reveals herpetic cervicitis. (From Oxman MN: Genital herpes. *In* Braude AI, Davis CE, Fierer J [eds]: Infectious Diseases and Medical Microbiology, ed 2. Philadelphia, WB Saunders, 1986, pp 1041–1054.

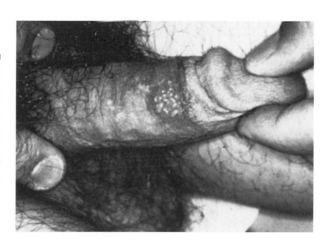

FIGURE 5–2

Recurrent genital herpes in the male patient. A typical patch of grouped vesicles on an erythematous base is seen on the shaft of the penis. (From Oxman MN: Genital herpes. *In* Braude AI, Davis CE, Fierer J [eds]: Infectious Diseases and Medical Microbiology, ed 2. Philadelphia, WB Saunders, 1986, pp 1041–1054.)

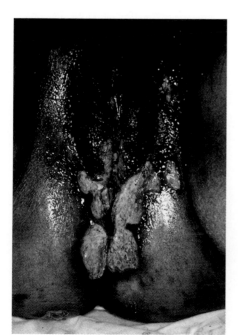

FIGURE 5–3

Primary herpes simplex virus infection in the perineum. Areas of erosion are extensive. Cultures are positive at this stage. Healing may take weeks with such extensive disease.

VENEREAL WARTS

TABLE 5–2

Types of Human Papillomaviruses

TYPE	SOURCE
HPV-1, -4	Plantar warts
HPV-2, -27, -29	Verruca vulgaris
HPV-3, -10, -26, -28	Flat warts
HPV-5, -8, -9, -12, -14, -15, -17, -19 to -25	Epidermodysplasia verruciformis
HPV-6, -11, -42, -43, -44	Genital warts and laryngeal papillomas
HPV-7	Butcher's warts
HPV-13, -32	Oral focal epithelial hyperplasia
HPV-16, -18, -30, -31, -33, -35, -39, -45, -51, -52, -56	Cervical dysplasia and carcinoma, bowenoid papulosis
HPV-30, -40	Laryngeal carcinoma

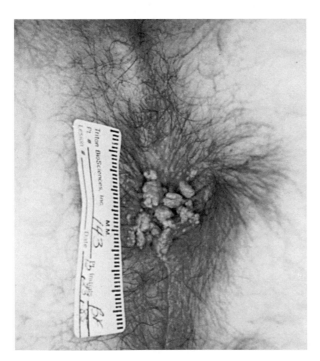

FIGURE 5–4

Genital warts involving the perianal region.

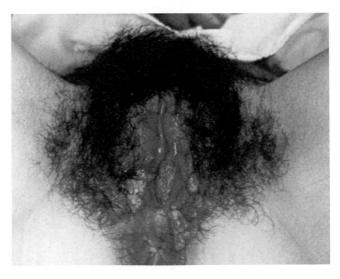

FIGURE 5–5

Genital warts involving the labia.

SYPHILIS

TABLE 5–3

Clinical Manifestations of Syphilis by Stages*

PRIMARY	SECONDARY	TERTIARY
Chancre on penis, labia, vagina, cervix, anus, rectum, lips, mouth, nipple, navel, finger Inguinal lymphadenopathy Condyloma latum†	Rash Condyloma latum Lymphadenopathy Hepatitis (subclinical) Systemic: fever, malaise, weight loss Neurologic: headache, meningismus, meningitis, cranial nerve disorders (optic neuritis, deafness, otitis), cerebrovascular accident Periostitis Uveitis, iritis Glomerulonephritis Arthritis	Benign late syphilis (gummata) of skin, subcutaneous tissues, bones, testis, liver Aortitis, aortic aneurysm Neurosyphilis: tabes dorsalis, paresis, psychosis, dementia, meningitis, cerebrovascular accident, spinal cord disease

*Early neurosyphilis, as seen in HIV-infected persons, is specifically not included in this table (see text).
†Most commonly an extension from a primary lesion, this condition may precede the onset of secondary (disseminated) syphilis, in which case it represents a stage intermediate between primary and secondary disease. Less frequently, condyloma latum appears in intertriginous areas during secondary (disseminated) infection.

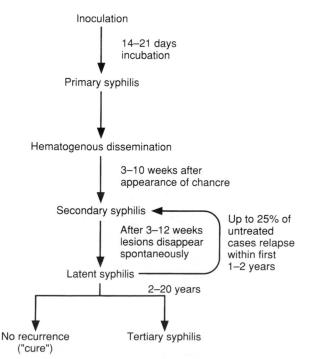

FIGURE 5–6

Time course of untreated syphilis. Treatment at any stage with accepted doses of penicillin nearly always eliminates disease (exceptions are late manifestations of tertiary syphilis and immunologic compromise caused by HIV infection).

FIGURE 5–7

Typical syphilitic chancre with clearly demarcated, slightly indurated margin and nonpurulent base.

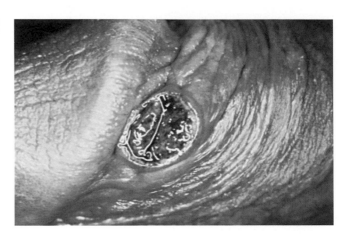

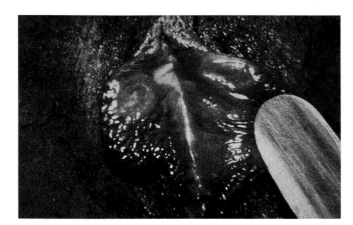

FIGURE 5–8

Primary syphilis. Typical appearance and location of chancre on the labia. This painless lesion in the female may not be readily visible on cursory examination.

FIGURE 5–9

Secondary syphilis. Highly infectious mucus patch on the base of the tongue.

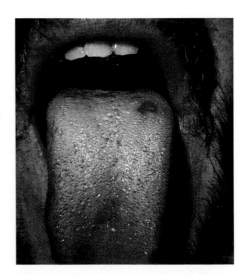

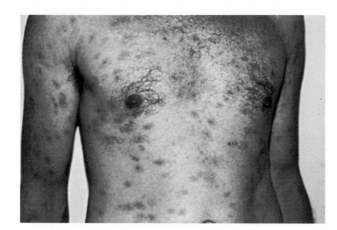

FIGURE 5–10

Typical generalized rash of secondary syphilis.

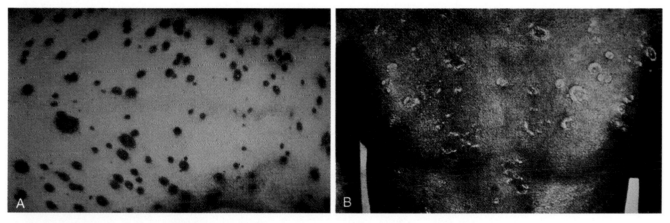

Less typical skin manifestations of secondary syphilis. Rash associated with syphilis has been described as macular, papular, or pustular.

FIGURE 5–11

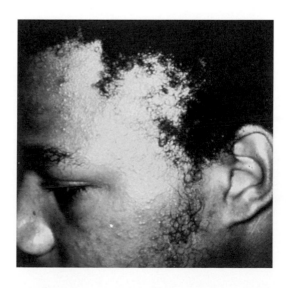

FIGURE 5–12

Alopecia associated with secondary syphilis. (Slide provided by Dr. John Knox.)

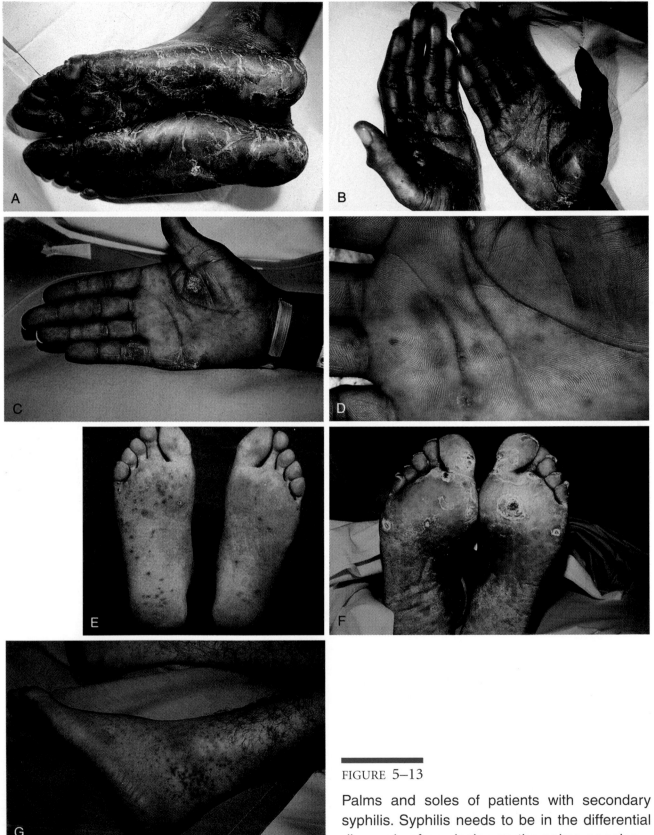

FIGURE 5–13

Palms and soles of patients with secondary syphilis. Syphilis needs to be in the differential diagnosis of any lesion on the palms or soles.

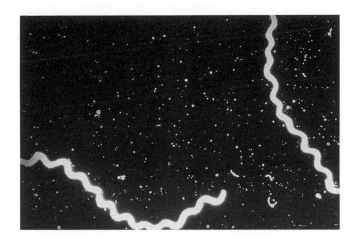

FIGURE 5–14

Darkfield microscopy of *Treponema pallidium*.

LYMPHOGRANULOMA VENEREUM AND CHANCROID

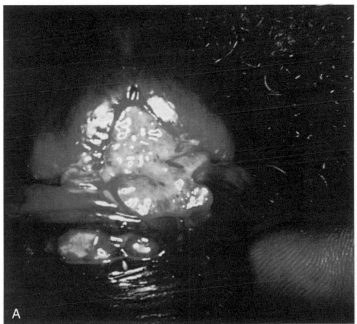

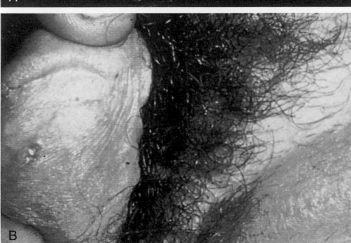

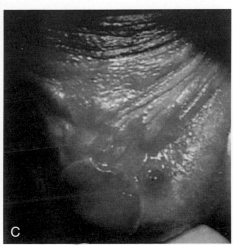

FIGURE 5–15

Genital ulcers. **A,** The eroded purulent ulcer of chancroid is painful and may be associated with painful inguinal adenitis. **B,** Lymphogranuloma venereum has a small, transient genital ulcer with swollen, extremely painful inguinal lymph nodes. **C,** The genital lesions of GI are painless, beefy red, raised lesions. (*C* from Al-Harmozi SA, el-Tonsy MH: Granuloma inguinale. Report of the first case in Qatar. Sex Transm Dis 13: 102, 1986.)

NEISSERIA GONORRHOEAE

TABLE 5–4

Clinical Presentations of Gonorrhea

Neonates
Asymptomatic mucosal infection
Conjunctivitis
Disseminated gonococcal infection

Men
Asymptomatic mucosal infection
Urethritis
Proctitis
Pharyngitis
Epididymitis
Disseminated gonococcal infection

Women
Asymptomatic mucosal infection
Cervicitis
Urethritis
Proctitis
Pharyngitis
Skene or Bartholin gland infection
Pelvic inflammatory disease
  (endometritis, salpingitis,
  peritonitis)
Disseminated gonococcal infection

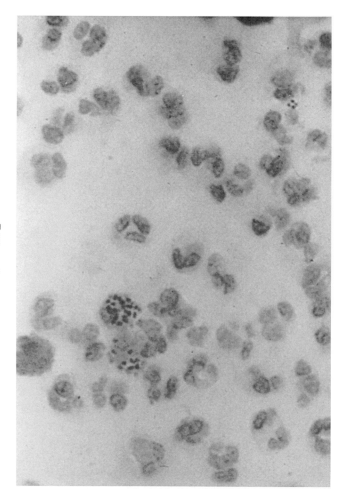

FIGURE 5–16

Urethral exudate with gram-negative diplococci.

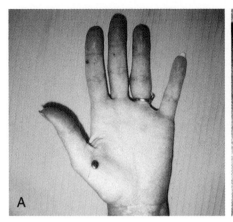
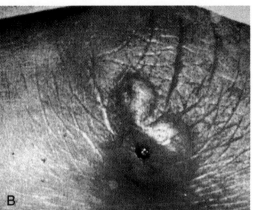

FIGURE 5–17

Skin lesions of disseminated gonococcal infection. **A,** Hemorrhagic pustule. **B,** Bullae that have yet to become hemorrhagic.

FIGURE 5–18

Septic arthritis. Patient has gonococcemia. Tenosynovitis and monoarticular arthritis in a sexually active patient must be considered to be gonococcal until proven otherwise.

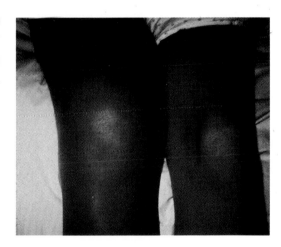

FIGURE 5–19

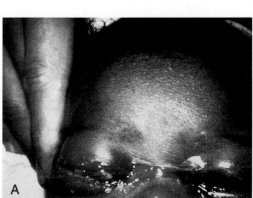
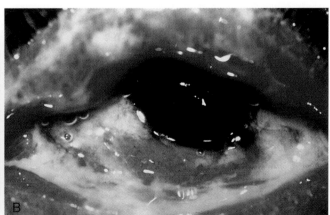

Gonococcal conjunctivitis. Neonate to whom conjunctivitis was transmitted at the time of birth.

PELVIC INFLAMMATORY DISEASE

TABLE 5–5

Bacteria Recovered from Upper Genital Tract of 188 Women
Hospitalized with Acute Pelvic Inflammatory Disease

BACTERIA	NUMBER OF ISOLATES
Anaerobes	
Prevotella sp.	88
Prevotella bivia	72
Prevotella disiens	25
Bacteroides sp.	99
Peptostreptococcus asaccharolyticus	93
Peptostreptococcus anaerobius	72
Facultative Bacteria	
Gardnerella vaginalis	121
Escherichia coli	25
Group B streptococcus	29
α-Hemolytic streptococcus	45
Nonhemolytic streptococcus	49
Coagulase-negative staphylococcus	72

From Sweet RL: Role of bacterial vaginosis in pelvic inflammatory disease. Clin Infect Dis 20(Suppl
2):S271–S275, 1995. © by University of Chicago.

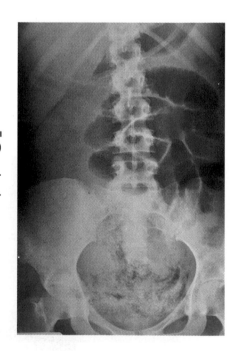

FIGURE 5–20

Uterine gas gangrene caused by *Clostridium perfringens.* Irregular linear collections of gas are present in the uterus. With the control of unsterile abortions, the incidence of this infection has decreased.

6

AIDS

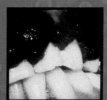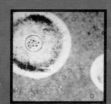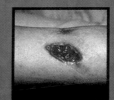

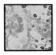

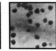

Over the last 15 years the AIDS epidemic has unfolded. Manifestations of rare diseases have now become commonplace, and new syndromes have been described.

ORAL MANIFESTATIONS

Observing the oral cavity in patients with human immunodeficiency virus (HIV) is an excellent way to assess the status of the immune system. Oral candidiasis is present only when cell-mediated immunity is significantly depressed. Gingivitis is common in patients with depressed CD4 counts. Kaposi's sarcoma may be manifested initially in the mouth. Aphthous ulcers can be recurrent and cause severe morbidity with intense pain and weight loss. Hairy leukoplakia is a surrogate marker that correlates to a rapid progression to AIDS.

FIGURE 6–1

Palatal petechiae in a patient with acute retroviral syndrome. The importance of an early diagnosis cannot be underestimated because treatment at this stage may be beneficial.

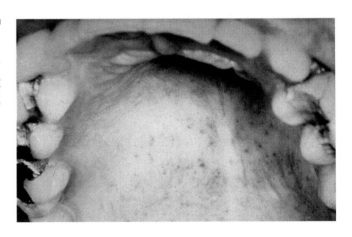

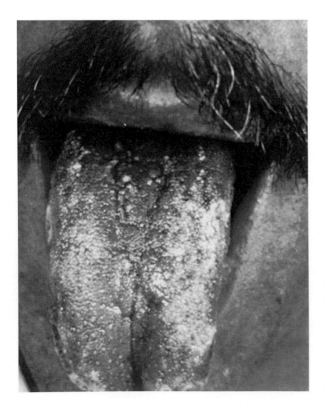

FIGURE 6–2

Candidiasis. Whitish, curdlike exudates on mucous membranes that are easily scraped off with a tongue depressor are characteristic of candidiasis. This is often associated with candidal esophagitis, which may result in severe dysphagia.

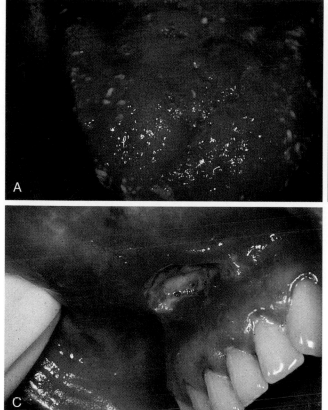

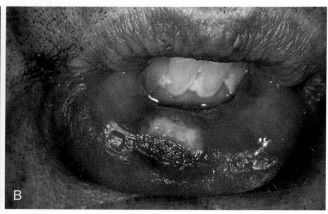

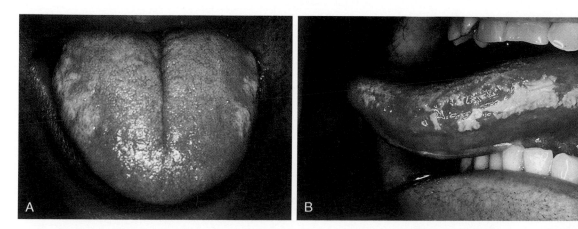

FIGURE 6–3

Aphthous ulcers are often multiple, very large, long-lasting, and recurrent. These ulcers are painful and can lead to weight loss. The differential includes herpes simplex virus (HSV), cytomegalovirus (CMV), and lymphoma. (Courtesy of Dr. Athena Pappas, Tufts University School of Dental Medicine, Boston, Massachusetts.)

Hairy leukoplakia. Note the raised lesions on the lateral aspects of the tongue. On cursory evaluation of the oropharynx these lesions may be missed or confused with thrush.

FIGURE 6–4

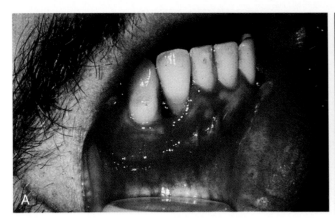
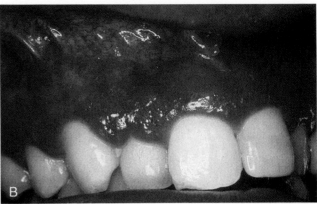

FIGURE 6–5

Gingivitis. This mixed infection of the gingiva is seen commonly in HIV and AIDS. It is recognized when patients describe bleeding during brushing and flossing of the teeth. Chronic infections can lead to loss of teeth. (Courtesy of Dr. Athena Pappas, Tufts University School of Dental Medicine, Boston, Massachusetts.)

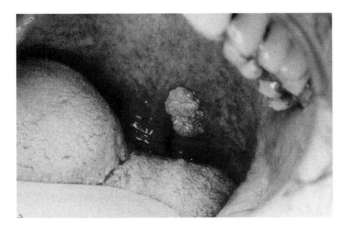

FIGURE 6–6

Papillomavirus. Typical warts occasionally are found in the oral cavity in patients with HIV. (Courtesy of Dr. Athena Pappas, Tufts University School of Dental Medicine, Boston, Massachusetts.)

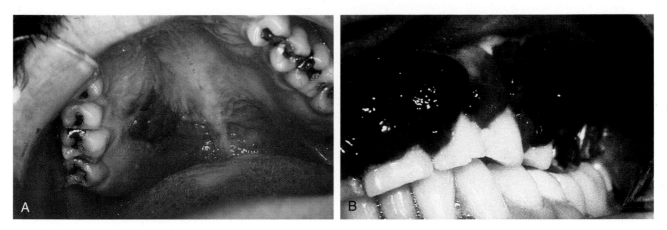

Kaposi's sarcoma. Small lesions on the hard palate may rapidly progress to include the gum surfaces.

FIGURE 6–7

FIGURE 6–8

Biopsy of this aphthouslike ulcer revealed primary lymphoma.

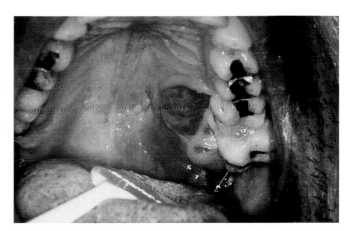

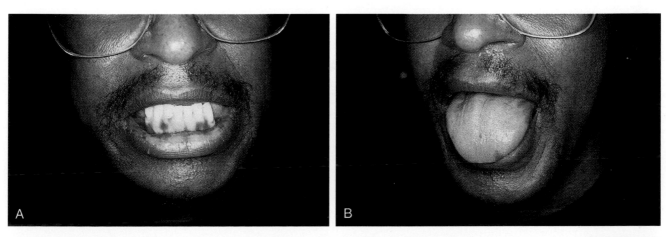

Hyperpigmentation of the gums and tongue developed in this patient 1 month after zidovudine therapy was begun.

FIGURE 6–9

SKIN/SOFT TISSUE MANIFESTATIONS

A number of opportunistic organisms may appear on the skin or subcutaneous tissues. Skin lesions may be the first manifestation of HIV infection in many patients. It is important to recognize these lesions and search for them on routine physical examination of patients with HIV.

TABLE 6–1

Common Cutaneous Infections That Provide Clues to Human Immunodeficiency Virus Infection

CUTANEOUS INFECTION	CLUE
Herpes simplex	Ulcerative lesion(s), lasting >1 mo, especially perianal location
Herpes zoster	Involvement of more than one dermatome; recurrent episodes
Verrucae	Multiple periungual lesions; numerous flat warts on face and beard area
Molluscum contagiosum	Multiple lesions on face, especially periorbital location; giant lesions
Impetigo	Axillary, inguinal, or other intertriginous locations
Staphylococcal folliculitis	Plaquelike folliculitis; progression to botryomycosis
Scabies	Hyperkeratotic crusted lesions (Norwegian scabies)
Oral candidiasis	Refractory or recurrent disease
Onychomycosis	Proximal white subungual involvement
Tinea versicolor	Extensive disease

TABLE 6–2

AIDS-Defining Cutaneous Disorders

Chronic herpes simplex ulceration >1 mo duration
Kaposi's sarcoma
Cutaneous cytomegalovirus infection, ulceration
Cutaneous cryptococcosis
Cutaneous lesions secondary to disseminated histoplasmosis, coccidioido-mycosis, or mycobacterial infections

TABLE 6–3

Relationship of Cutaneous Infections to CD4+ Cell Count

CUTANEOUS DISEASE	AVERAGE CD4+ CELL COUNT AT DISEASE PRESENTATION (CELLS/mm^3)
Acute exanthem of HIV	Normal
Bacterial folliculitis impetigo	>500
Tinea	>500
Seborrheic dermatitis	>500
Intraepithelial neoplasia	<500
Oral hairy leukoplakia	<400
Verrucae	500–250
Herpes zoster	500–250
Herpes simplex	500–250
Scabies	<250
Bacillary angiomatosis	<250
Leishmaniasis	<250
Molluscum contagiosum	<250
Oral candidiasis	<250
Cytomegalovirus infection	<200

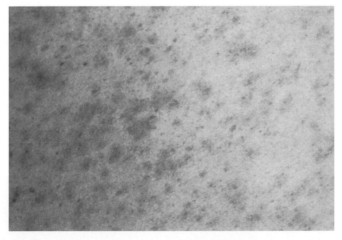

FIGURE 6–10

Acute exanthem of HIV infection. A widespread eruption of fine macules and papules distributed over the trunk, extremities, and sometimes the head and neck is characteristic of the viral exanthem of HIV infection. This eruption is seen only rarely and may be confused with other viral exanthems. It is imperative that any patient with the acute retroviral syndrome be seen as soon as possible for consideration of initiating of antiviral medications. The differential diagnosis includes enterovirus, adenovirus, CMV, and Epstein-Barr virus.

FIGURE 6–11

Bacillary angiomatosis. These small red-purple papules are caused by infection with *Bartonella henselae* or *Bartonella quintana*. The organisms are seen on a Warthin-Starry stain. Prior to the AIDS epidemic, this syndrome was not recognized. Patients with HIV who own cats should be advised to call their doctor should such lesions appear.

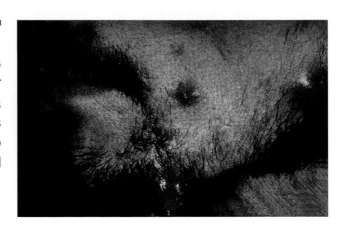

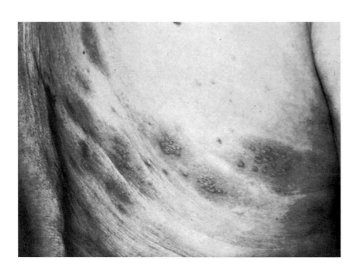

FIGURE 6–12

Herpes zoster. A linear dermatomal distribution of painful vesicles on erythematous bases is characteristic of herpes zoster. This may be the presenting manifestation of HIV infection and, when present in the proper clinical context, should cause the clinician to perform an HIV test.

FIGURE 6–13

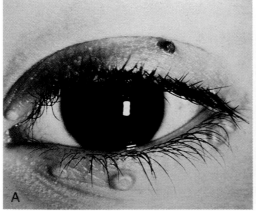

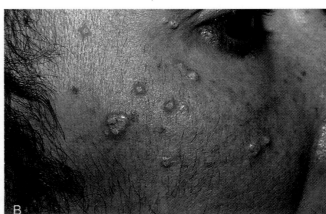

Molluscum contagiosum. Multiple lesions are seen on the face of people infected with HIV.

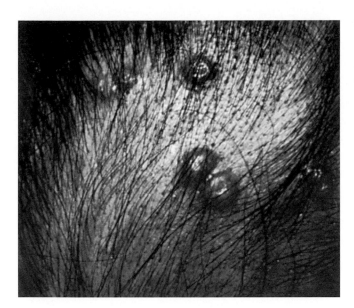

FIGURE 6–14

Atypical mycobacterial infection. Two draining ulcerations caused by *Mycobacterium avium-intracellulare.* Biopsies and cultures are essential to establish such diagnoses.

FIGURE 6–15

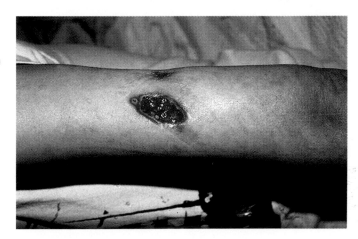

Mycobacterium haemophilum. This patient with AIDS presented with a disseminated mycobacterial infection. Biopsy cultures of the skin lesions revealed *Mycobacterium haemophilum.* The patient did well with therapy, and the lesions rapidly resolved.

FIGURE 6–16

Cutaneous cryptococcosis. This somewhat yellowish translucent crusted papule with a nondescript appearance was caused by *Cryptococcus neoformans.* This emphasizes the need to take biopsy specimens and cultures of virtually any lesion in a patient with HIV infection and fever.

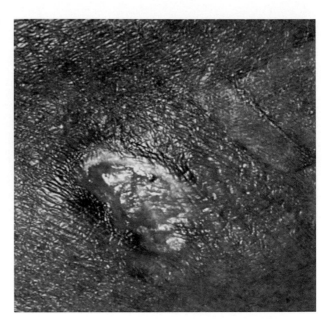

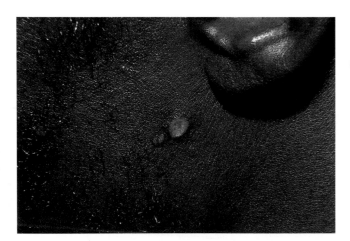

FIGURE 6–17

Cryptococcus neoformans. Nodular or ulcerative skin lesions are seen in disseminated disease. In AIDS patients, meningeal findings may be minimal, and patients often present with a fever of unknown origin. Biopsy of the lesions reveals encapsulated organisms.

FIGURE 6–18

Histoplasmosis. This HIV-infected trucker spent much time in the Midwest. He presented with fevers and plaquelike lesions that grew *Histoplasma capsulatum* on biopsy.

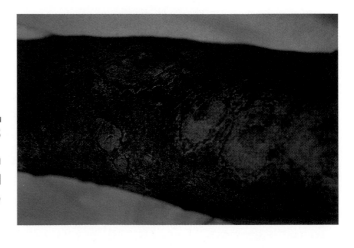

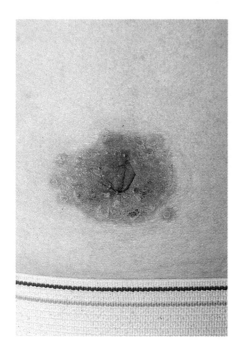

FIGURE 6–19

Cutaneous candidal infection. This patient with advanced AIDS has superficial candidal infection in the periumbilical region.

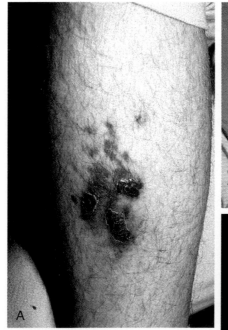

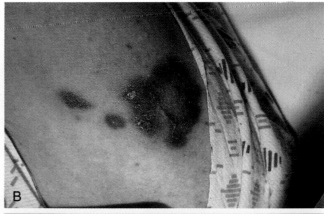

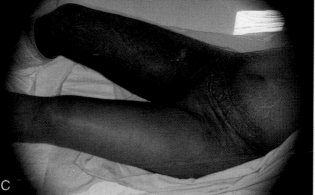

FIGURE 6–20

Kaposi's sarcoma. Lesions can be nodular, plaquelike, and extensive. All three patients had AIDS. Human herpesvirus type 8 has been implicated in the pathogenesis of this tumor.

FIGURE 6–21

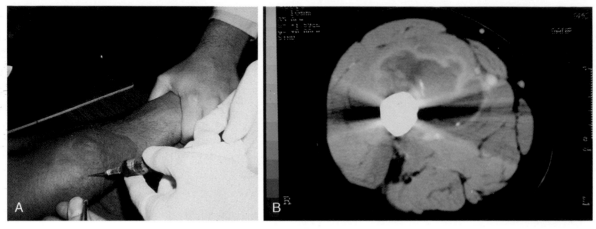

Pyomyositis. This disease, which was known in the tropics, has become common in persons with HIV infection. Patients present with pain and fever, and at times the diagnosis may not be apparent. Computed tomography (CT) scans are used to determine the extent of disease. *Staphylococcus aureus* is the most common isolate.

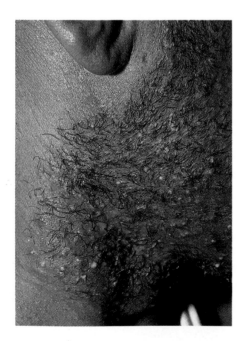

FIGURE 6–22

Folliculitis. Chronic folliculitis has been described with HIV infection. The condition can be caused by pyogenic bacteria or fungi, as in this case.

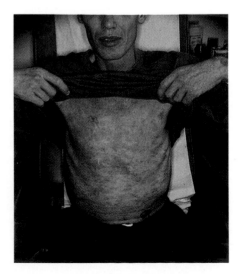

FIGURE 6–23

Psoriasis. Chronic skin disorders such as psoriasis may be extensive and debilitating in patients with AIDS. Dyshidrosis may exacerbate the underlying condition.

NEUROLOGIC MANIFESTATIONS

Because of the inability of many antiviral agents to penetrate in high concentration into the central nervous system (CNS), signs of dementia arise in many patients with late stage disease. Today, hospitalized patients with AIDS often have CNS manifestations of HIV or opportunistic illnesses such as toxoplasmosis, lymphoma (EBV), CMV, or progressive multifocal leukoencephalopathy (PML). Obtaining a CT scan in patients with neurologic manifestations may help with the diagnosis; however, brain biopsy is still the gold standard for most lesions that do not respond to antitoxoplasmosis medications.

TABLE 6–4

Etiology of Neuropathic Syndromes in Human Immunodeficiency Virus Infection

Immune-mediated Response to Human Immunodeficiency Virus Bell palsy Acute inflammatory demyelinating neuropathy (Guillain-Barré syndrome) Chronic inflammatory demyelinating neuropathy	**Meningitis** Cryptococcal Neurosyphilitic Tuberculous
Vasculitis Bell palsy Ataxic dorsal radiculopathy Mononeuritis multiplex: hepatitis B virus–associated cryoglobulinemia	**Malignant Neoplasm** Lymphoma **Nutritional Deficiencies** Multiple vitamin deficiencies: folate, pyridoxine Vitamin B_{12} deficiency
Opportunistic Invasive Herpesvirus Infections Cytomegalovirus Polyradiculopathy Multiple mononeuropathy Herpes simplex virus Polyradiculopathy Varicella-zoster virus Herpes zoster Polyradiculopathy	**Drug Toxicity from Concurrent Antiinfectives** Antiretroviral nucleoside analogs Dideoxycytidine Dideoxyinosine Stavudine Niacin analogs: isoniazid **Idiopathic Neuropathy** Predominantly sensory neuropathy of acquired immunodeficiency syndrome

FIGURE 6–24

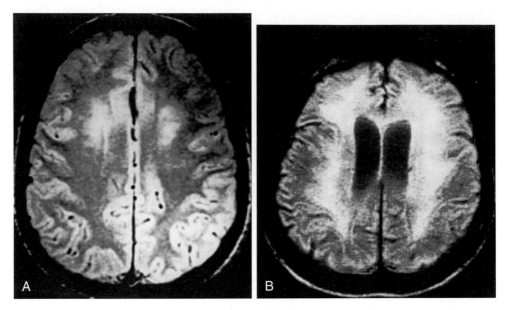

HIV-1 Encephalopathy (HIVE). **A,** Magnetic resonance imaging (MRI) scan (T2-weighted image) from a 33-year-old homosexual man, showing large areas of abnormal signal intensity in the white matter. No mass effect is present. **B,** MRI scan (T2-weighted image) from a 38-year-old bisexual man with late HIVE demonstrating enlargement of the ventricles, cerebral atrophy, and diffuse abnormalities throughout the white matter.

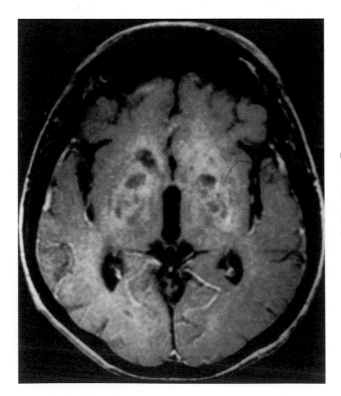

FIGURE 6–25

MRI scan in cryptococcal meningitis showing discrete areas of low density in basal ganglia representing cryptococcomas.

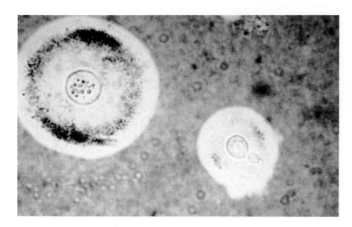

FIGURE 6-26

Cryptococcus. India ink slide shows the large capsule around the organisms present in the cerebrospinal fluid (CSF) of this patient with AIDS.

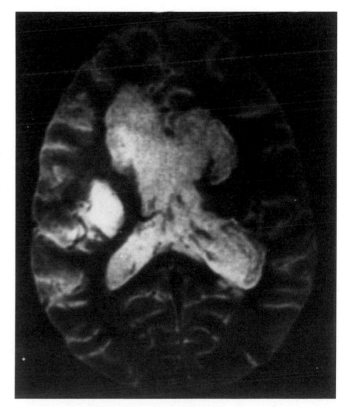

FIGURE 6-27

CMV encephalitis. Cranial MRI scan of fulminant CMV encephalitis showing prominent inflammation in ependymal and periventricular area.

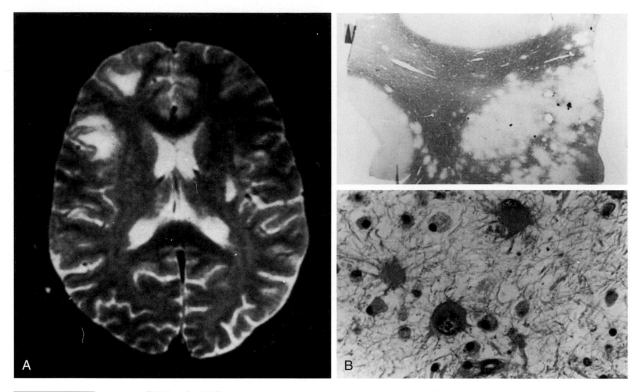

FIGURE 6–28   PML. **A,** MRI scan showing multiple areas of hyperintensity confined to the subcortical white matter in the frontoparietal area. No mass effect and no enhancement with contrast medium are seen. **B,** Luxol fast blue stain of brain showing multiple demyelinative foci. High power shows transformed bizarre-looking astrocytes and inclusion-bearing oligodendrocytes.

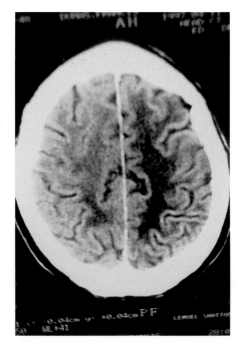

FIGURE 6–29

PML. Extensive disease is noted in patient with AIDS. Despite no adequate therapy for the JC virus, the patient has done well on HAART therapy.

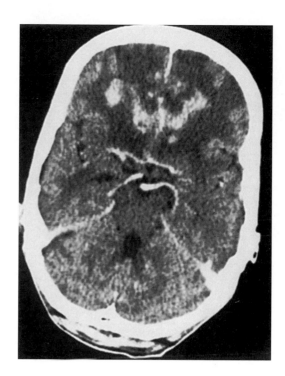

FIGURE 6–30

Primary CNS lymphoma. CT scan from a patient with autopsy-proven primary CNS lymphoma. There is a multicentric contrast-enhanced lesion in the frontal lobes with massive surrounding edema and posterior displacement of the middle cerebral arteries.

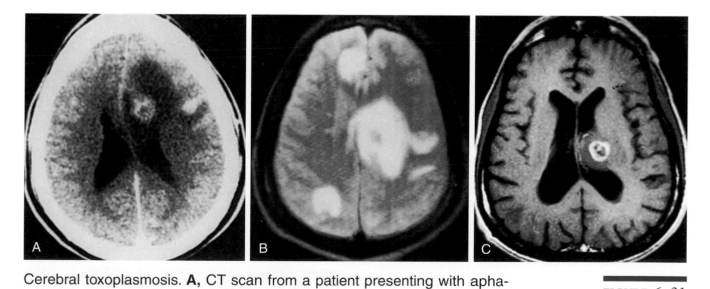

Cerebral toxoplasmosis. **A,** CT scan from a patient presenting with aphasia and hemiparesis demonstrating several contrast-enhanced lesions. Surrounding edema and a significant mass effect with displacement of midline structures are seen. With treatment, the patient had a normal CT scan. **B,** MRI scan (T2-weighted image) from the patient in *A* obtained at the same time *A* was obtained, showing the ability of this imaging technique to demonstrate occipital lesions not seen on the CT scan. **C,** MRI scan with gadolinium showing enhancement in basal ganglion and mass effect.

FIGURE 6–31

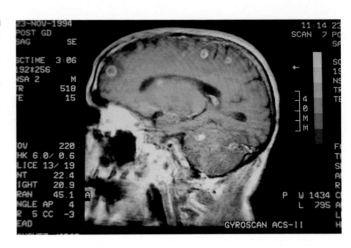

FIGURE 6–32

CNS toxoplasmosis. Sagittal view of MRI scan. Multiple lesions are characteristic of toxoplasmosis. Following 3 weeks of antitoxoplasmosis medications, many of the lesions markedly resolved.

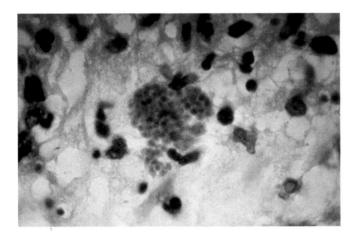

FIGURE 6–33

Toxoplasmosis. A brain biopsy specimen clearly shows tachyzoites.

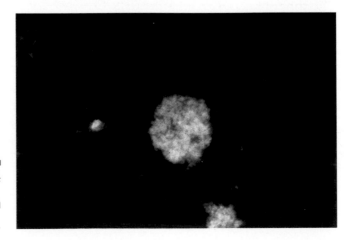

FIGURE 6–34

Immunofluorescent staining of a touch preparation from brain tissue in a patient with CNS toxoplasmosis.

GASTROINTESTINAL MANIFESTATIONS

Diarrhea and chronic wasting syndrome remain major problems in persons with HIV infection. In addition, AIDS cholangiopathy can cause severe morbidity in late stage disease. An array of organisms from viruses to protozoa can infect cells within the gastrointestinal tract. Biopsies are needed to confirm the diagnosis in many instances.

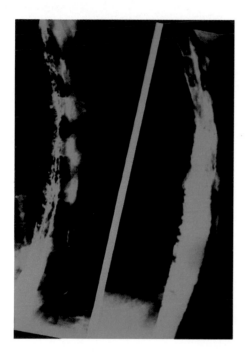

FIGURE 6–35

Ragged mucosal surface is seen in the barium swallow of a patient with AIDS and odynophagia. Subsequent biopsy revealed candidiasis.

FIGURE 6–36

Esophageal *Candida* endoscopy. White plaques confirm the diagnosis of *Candida* esophagitis.

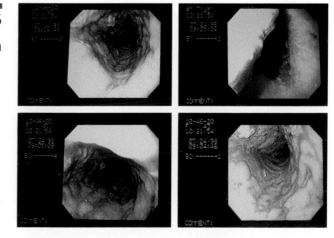

FIGURE 6–37

Histologic specimen demonstrating *Candida* esophagitis.

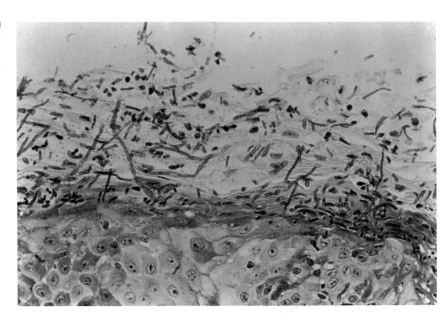

TABLE 6–5

Prevalence of Enteric Pathogens in Patients with Acquired Immunodeficiency Syndrome with Diarrhea

PATHOGEN	MEAN (%)	RANGE (%)
Cryptosporidium	20	7–37
Microsporida	19	2–39
Cytomegalovirus	20	8–45
Mycobacterium avium	9	2–25
Giardia lamblia	5	2–12
Entamoeba histolytica	3	0–25
Campylobacter jejuni	3	0–11
Clostridium difficile	2	0–7
Salmonella sp.	2	0–25
Shigella	2	0–5
Isospora	1	0–4
Enteric viruses	4	2–10

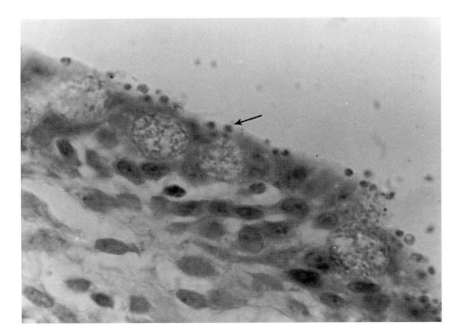

FIGURE 6–38

Cryptosporidia *(arrow)* studding the small bowel epithelial surface of a patient with AIDS. (Giemsa stain, × 450.)

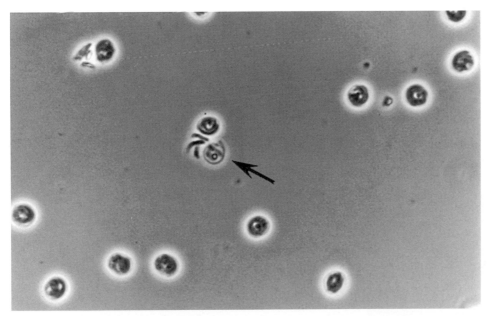

FIGURE 6–39

Human stool–derived *Cryptosporidium* oocysts. Excysting oocyst *(arrow)* is releasing three of its four sporozoites. (Phase-contrast microscopy × 630.)

FIGURE 6–40

Cryptosporidium. This 18-year-old patient with AIDS produced over 7 L of watery stool a day. Abundant *Cryptosporidium* organisms can be seen in this modified Ziehl-Neelsen stain. (Courtesy of Dr. David Hamer, New England Medical Center, Boston, Massachusetts.)

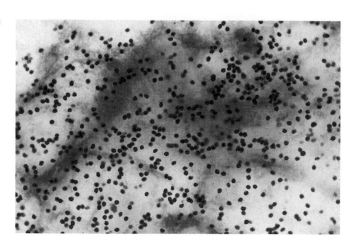

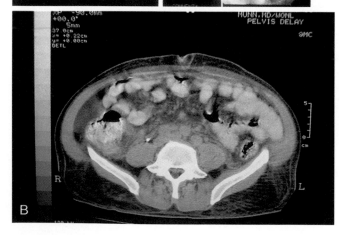

FIGURE 6–41

CMV colitis. Note the extensive ulcerations along the bowel mucosa. CT scan revealed marked bowel wall thickening, and biopsy was positive for CMV inclusions.

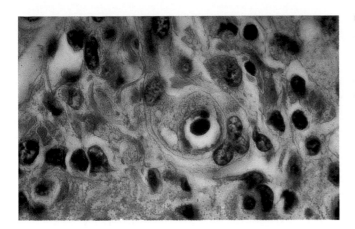

FIGURE 6–42

CMV hepatitis. Enlarged cells containing inclusions are present in this biopsy specimen from a patient with AIDS.

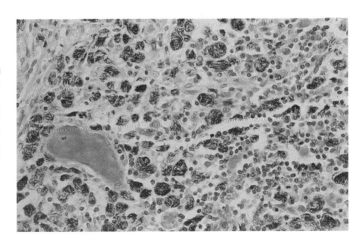

FIGURE 6–43

Mycobacterium avium complex–induced hepatitis. It is typical to see a large burden of organisms with a lack of organized granuloma formation in patients with AIDS.

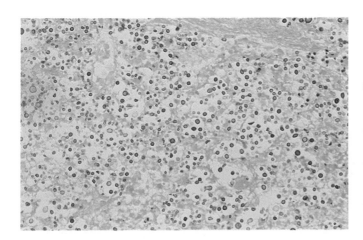

FIGURE 6–44

Autopsy specimen from the liver showing *Cryptococcus.* This patient had cryptococcal meningitis with a miliary pattern of disease on the chest radiograph. Despite full doses of amphotericin B and flucytosine (5-FC), the patient failed to respond clinically.

FIGURE 6–45

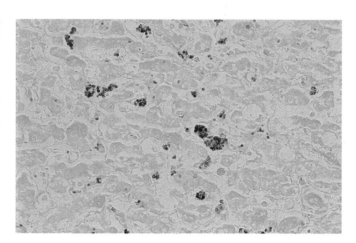

This patient with AIDS had disseminated histoplasmosis that produced a sepsis syndrome, which included disseminated intravascular coagulation. At autopsy, organisms are present throughout all the parenchymal organs including the liver.

PULMONARY MANIFESTATIONS

Pneumonia remains a major cause of morbidity and mortality in patients with HIV and AIDS. It is essential to obtain baseline chest radiographs in all new patients. Consideration of pneumonia is needed in any HIV-infected patient with a febrile illness, even if respiratory signs are lacking.

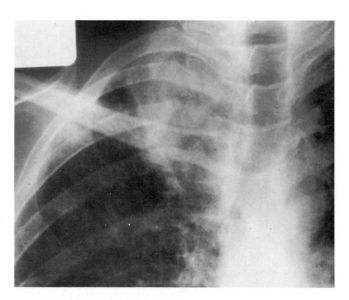

FIGURE 6–46

Detail of a frontal view chest radiograph shows a focal right upper lobe abnormality caused by *P. carinii.*

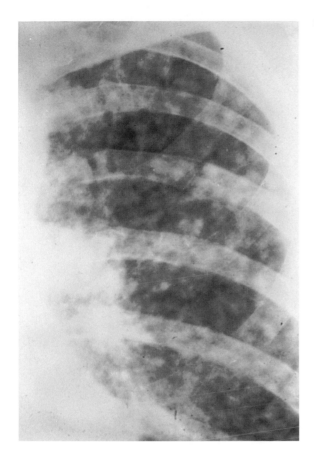

FIGURE 6–47

Detail of a frontal view chest radiograph shows a finely nodular (miliary) pattern of infiltration caused by *P. carinii.*

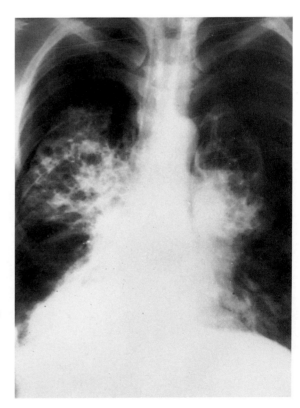

FIGURE 6–48

Chest radiograph showing bilateral spontaneous pneumothoraces and marked cystic changes in the lungs caused by *P. carinii.*

FIGURE 6–49

Cyst forms of *P. carinii* stained with the Gomori methenamine–silver nitrate method. The dark-staining cysts are 5 to 6 μm in diameter and are usually round or cup shaped. The intracystic sporozoites are not seen with this stain.

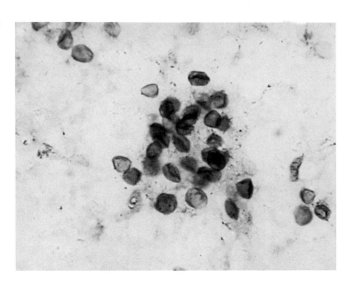

FIGURE 6–50

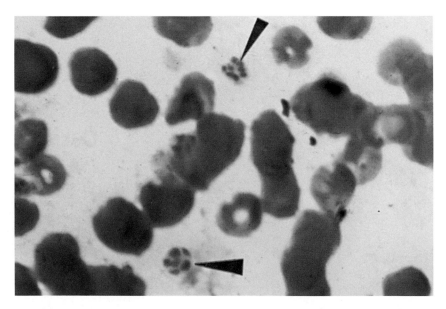

Imprint of lung biopsy specimen stained with Giemsa method. Clusters of *Pneumocystis carinii* sporozoites *(arrowheads)* are located within the cyst. The cyst wall does not stain, but an area of rarefaction is usually discernible.

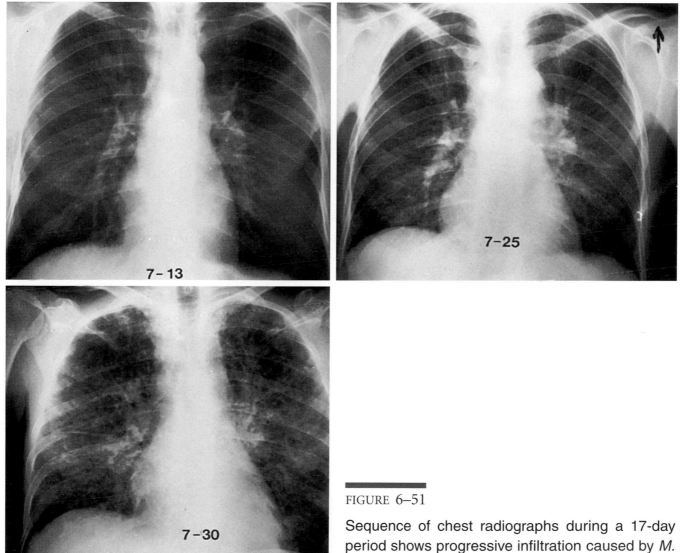

FIGURE 6–51

Sequence of chest radiographs during a 17-day period shows progressive infiltration caused by *M. tuberculosis* in an AIDS patient.

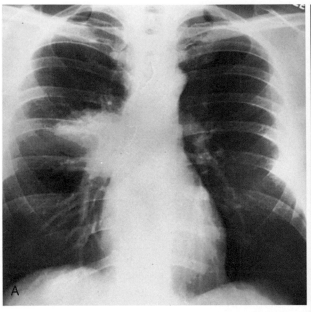

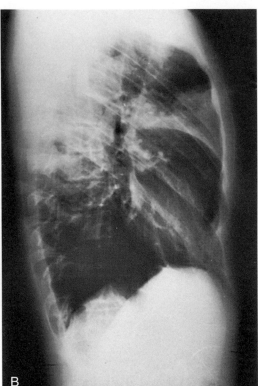

FIGURE 6–52

Frontal **(A)** and lateral **(B)** chest radiographs show an infiltration in the anterior segment of the right upper lobe caused by *M. avium* complex.

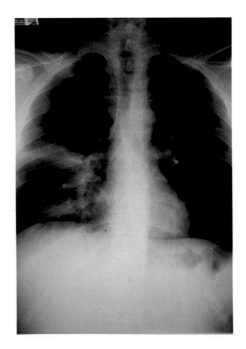

FIGURE 6–53

Kaposi's sarcoma (KS) of the lung. With KS the viscera and frequently the lung may be involved. Mass lesions are usually present, and effusions may be large. This patient with cutaneous KS has a nodule in the right lung.

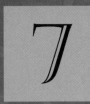

INFECTIONS
OF THE
SKIN AND
SOFT TISSUE

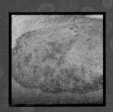
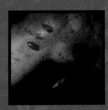
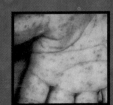

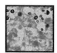
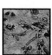
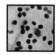

Recognition of skin and soft tissue infections is important at an early stage so appropriate treatment can be initiated. The shorter the time lapse from the infection's inception until antibiotics are begun or until surgical debridement is done the better the prognosis. It is important to consider underlying risk factors associated with a skin and soft tissue infection (e.g., underlying skin condition, foreign body) and the most likely pathogens (e.g., *Staphylococcus aureus* in an intensive care unit patient or *Pasteurella* in a patient who has been bitten by a dog).

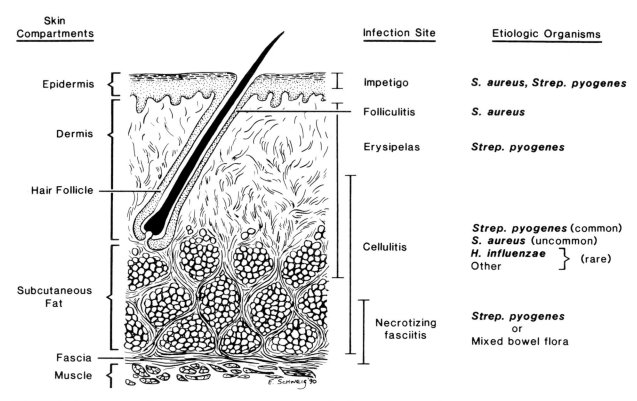

Skin Compartments		Infection Site	Etiologic Organisms
Epidermis		Impetigo	*S. aureus, Strep. pyogenes*
Dermis		Folliculitis	*S. aureus*
		Erysipelas	*Strep. pyogenes*
Hair Follicle			
		Cellulitis	*Strep. pyogenes* (common) *S. aureus* (uncommon) *H. influenzae* } (rare) Other
Subcutaneous Fat			
		Necrotizing fasciitis	*Strep. pyogenes* or Mixed bowel flora
Fascia			
Muscle			

FIGURE 7–1 Cutaneous anatomy, sites of infection, and infecting organisms.

TABLE 7–1

Some Considerations in Managing Bacterial Skin and Soft Tissue Infections

Primary versus secondary
Infection portal of entry
Impaired host defenses against infection
Associated signs and symptoms
Localization and morphology of lesion
Recent environmental exposure

TABLE 7–2

Resident Cutaneous Flora and Associated Skin Disorders

ORGANISMS	ASSOCIATED CUTANEOUS DISORDER
Gram-Positive Cocci	
Staphylococcus aureus	Impetigo, ecthyma, blistering distal dactylitis, pustules, folliculitis, cutaneous abscesses
Coagulase-negative staphylococci	—
Micrococcus species	—
M. sedentarius	Pitted keratolysis
Gram-Positive Bacilli	
Corynebacterium species	Trichomycosis axillaris, dermatophytosis complex, axillary odor,
C. minutissimum	erythrasma, pitted keratolysis
Brevibacterium species	Cheesy foot odor
Propionibacterium species	—
P. acnes	Acne
Gram-Negative Bacilli	
Acinetobacter species	—
Fungl	
Pityrosporum orbiculare (ovale)	Tinea (pityriasis) versicolor
	Seborrheic dermatitis
	Pityrosporum folliculitis

FUNGAL INFECTIONS OF THE SKIN

Fungal infections of the skin span a wide spectrum of disease. The fungal infection may be superficial, locally invasive, or part of a systemic infection. With systemic disease, early recognition and initiation of appropriate antifungal agents may be life saving. All atypical skin lesions in a febrile patient should be considered for biopsy and culture.

TABLE 7–3

Summary of Deep Fungal Infections

DISEASE	CAUSATIVE ORGANISM	ENDEMIC AREA	DISTINCTIVE CUTANEOUS LESION(S)
Cryptococcosis	*Cryptococcus neoformans*	Widespread distribution; found in pigeon excrement	Cellulitis, purpura, molluscum contagiosum–like lesions
Histoplasmosis	*Histoplasma capsulatum*	Central river valleys of United States; in droppings of blackbirds	Acneiform lesions, oral ulcerations
Blastomycosis	*Blastomyces dermatitidis*	Southeastern and south-central North America	Raised plaque with heaped-up border; skin and mucosal ulcerations
Coccidioidomy-cosis	*Coccidioides immitis*	Lower Sonoran life zones	Verrucous plaques, erythema nodosum
Sporotrichosis	*Sporothrix schenckii*	Tropical or subtropical Americas; found in soil and wood	Linear nodules in line of lymphatic drainage
Paracoccidio-idomycosis	*Paracoccidioides brasiliensis*	Latin America, from Mexico to Argentina	Mucosal ulceration, periorificial lesions

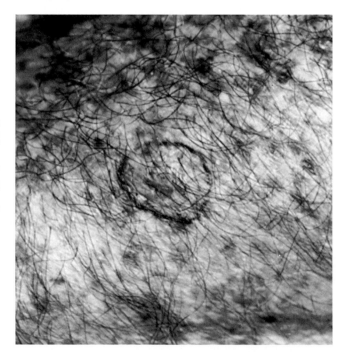

FIGURE 7–2

Early skin lesion of disseminated blastomycosis. A small papule is present on the forearm of a patient with systemic blastomycosis. (Courtesy of Dr. Corwin Dunn, Christ Hospital, Cincinnati, Ohio.)

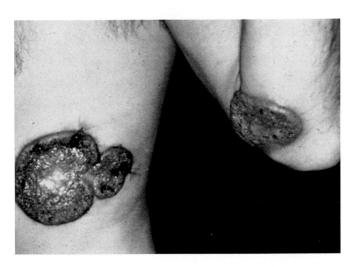

FIGURE 7–3

Advanced skin lesions of disseminated blastomycosis on the thorax and arm. The patient had an 18-month history of progressive skin disease. Note the verrucous borders and ulcerated center as well as the numerous black dots on the arm lesion.

FIGURE 7–4

Blastomyces yeast in potassium hydroxide preparation from skin aspiration. Note the broad-based budding of this fungal form.

FIGURE 7–5

Angular cheilitis and lip lesions caused by *Paracoccidioides brasiliensis*. Hemorrhagic spots are evident at both angles of the lips. (Courtesy of Angela Restrepo, PhD, Mycology Unit, Corporacion des Investigaciones Biológicas, Medellín, Colombia.)

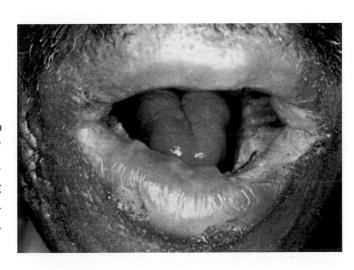

FIGURE 7–6

Large ulceration of the tongue caused by *Paracoc-cidioides.* Hemorrhagic spots are widely dispersed. (Courtesy of Angela Restrepo, PhD, Mycology Unit, Corporacion des Investigaciones Biológicas, Medel-lín, Colombia.)

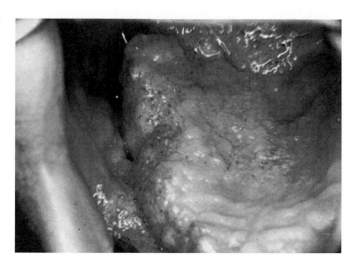

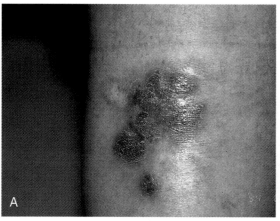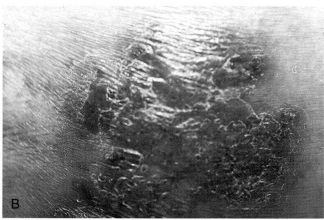

FIGURE 7–7

Chromoblastomycosis. **A,** Multiple plaques on the lower leg. **B,** Close-up of *A.* (Courtesy of Dr. Nellie Konnikov, New England Medical Center, Boston, Massachusetts.)

FIGURE 7–8

Chromoblastomycosis. Verrucous plaques on the lateral aspect of the foot.

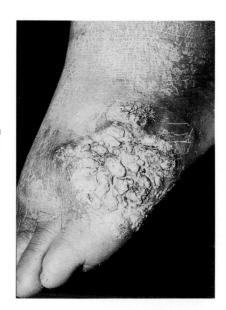

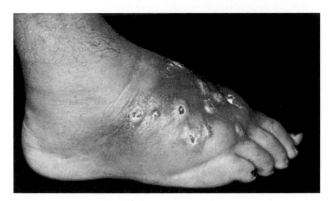

FIGURE 7–9

Mycetoma of the foot. (Courtesy of Dr. Victor Newcomer, Santa Monica, California.)

FIGURE 7–10

The chain of ulcerating, nodular skin lesions is typical of the cutaneous form of sporotrichosis. Characteristically, the older distal lesions show more ulceration and the younger proximal lesions have not yet broken down. The "bridges" of normal skin between lesions occur frequently, but a firm, swollen lymphatic "cord" connecting the nodules can be felt under the skin.

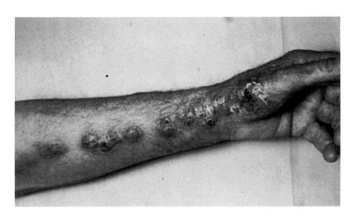

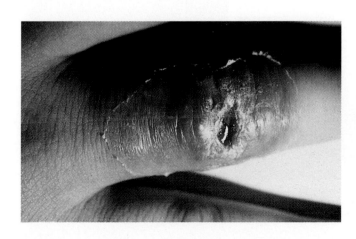

FIGURE 7–11

Sporothrix schenckii. Primary site of infection on the finger appears indurated with a nonhealing ulcer. (Courtesy of Dr. Mark Drapkin, Newton Wellesley Hospital, Newton, Massachusetts.)

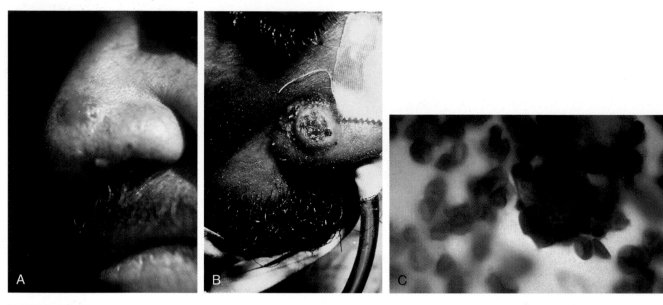

FIGURE 7–12

Coccidioides immitis. Skin lesions of hematogenous origin may appear as verrucous papules, plaques, or ulcers. The nose is frequently involved. The organism can be seen on Papanicolaou stain in scrapings of the ulcerative skin lesions. (*B* and *C* courtesy of Dr. Mark Drapkin, Newton Wellesley Hospital, Newton, Massachusetts.)

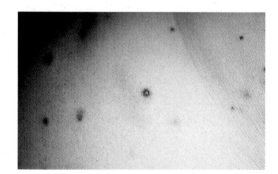

FIGURE 7–13

Candidal skin lesion. Pustules are seen as part of disseminated candidal infection. (Courtesy of Dr. Mark Drapkin, Newton Wellesley Hospital, Newton, Massachusetts.)

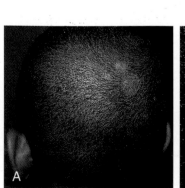
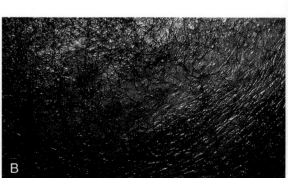
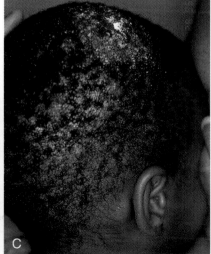

FIGURE 7–14

Tinea capitis. **A,** Multiple, scaly alopecic plaques. **B,** Black-dot tinea capitis. **C,** Kerion with visibly enlarged postauricular lymph node.

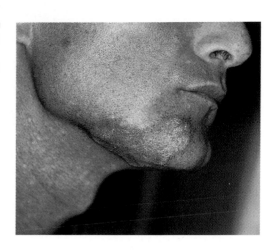

FIGURE 7–15

Tinea barbae. Pink scaly plaque with raised red border in the beard area.

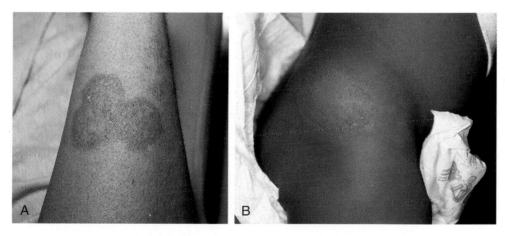

FIGURE 7–16

Tinea corporis. **A,** Coalescing scaly annular plaques on the forearm. **B,** Annular erythematous plaque on an infant's hip, occluded by the diaper.

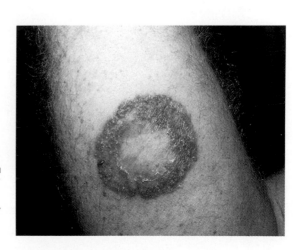

FIGURE 7–17

Tinea corporis. Inflammatory annular plaque with vesicular border on the forearm.

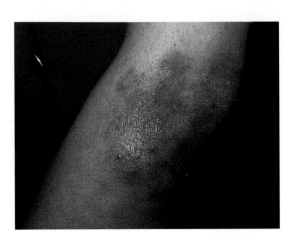

FIGURE 7–18

Majocchi granuloma. Coalescing plaques with follicular papules on the elbow.

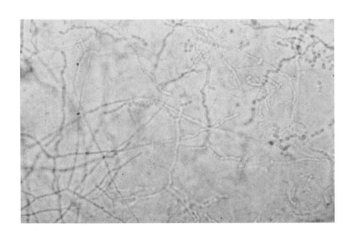

FIGURE 7–19

KOH preparation. Dermatophyte hyphae visualized on microscopic examination. (Courtesy of Dr. Victor New-comer, Santa Monica, California.)

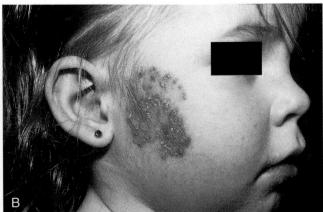

FIGURE 7–20

Tinea faciei. **A,** Erythematous annular plaque in the left preauricular area. Note the relative absence of scale. **B,** Inflammatory, erythematous, slightly scaly plaques and papules on the face of a 2-year-old girl.

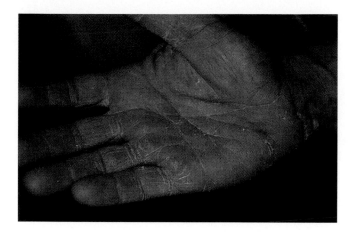

FIGURE 7–21

Tinea manuum. (Courtesy of Dr. Nellie Konnikov, New England Medical Center Hospital, Boston, Massachusetts.)

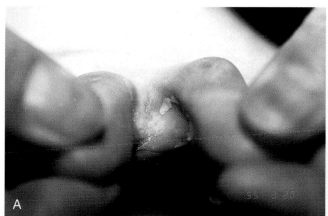
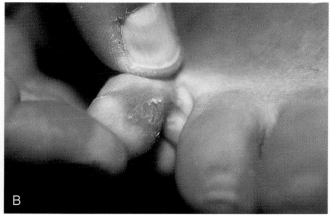

Tinea pedis. **A,** Interdigital maceration and scaling. **B,** Interdigital maceration and scaling. (*A* courtesy of Dr. Nellie Konnikov, New England Medical Center Hospital, Boston, Massachusetts.)

FIGURE 7–22

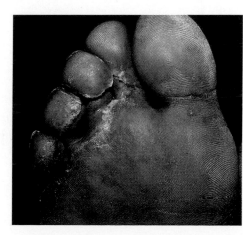

FIGURE 7–23

Dermatophytosis complex. Mixed infection with dermatophytes and bacteria.

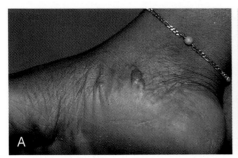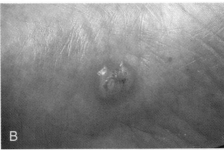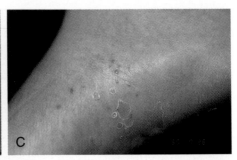

FIGURE 7–24

Vesicular tinea pedis. **A,** Scattered and coalescing vesicles. **B,** Coalescing vesicles. **C,** Multiple small vesicles and peeling collarettes.

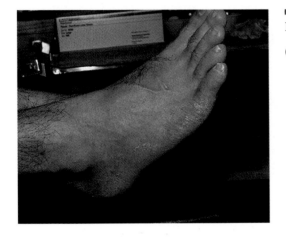

FIGURE 7–25

Chronic moccasintype tinea pedis.

FIGURE 7–26

Tinea incognito. Tinea corporis previously treated with hydrocortisone. Note the clinical similarity to tinea in an immunosuppressed patient with AIDS (see Fig. 7–34).

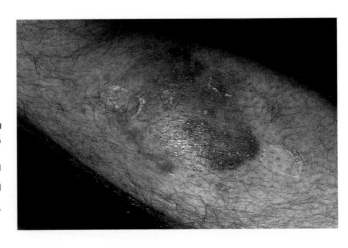

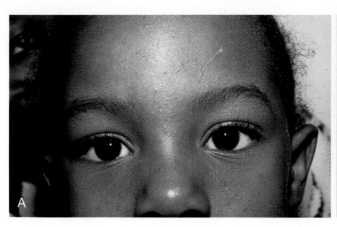 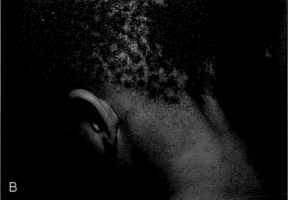

Dermatophytid or id reaction. **A,** Fine papular eruption on the face of a 3-year-old girl with tinea capitis. **B,** Tinea capitis with fine papular id reaction on the neck.

FIGURE 7–27

FIGURE 7–28

Onychomycosis in a patient with trisomy 21.

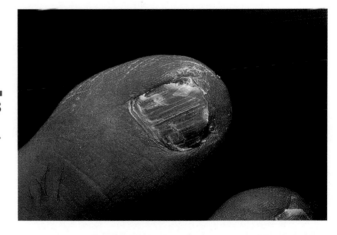

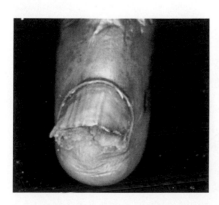

FIGURE 7–29

Distal subungual onychomycosis. Note the distal subungual hyper-keratosis.

FIGURE 7–30

Proximal subungual onychomycosis. This type of ony-chomycosis occurs more commonly in AIDS. (Courtesy of Dr. Nellie Konnikov, New England Medical Center Hospital, Boston, Massachusetts.)

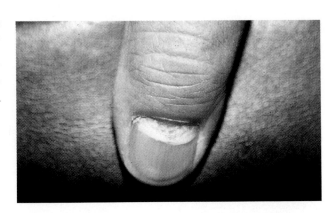

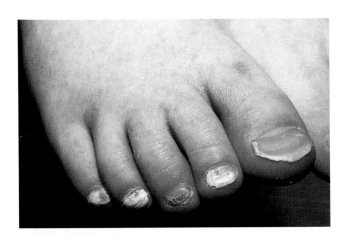

FIGURE 7–31

Superficial white onychomycosis.

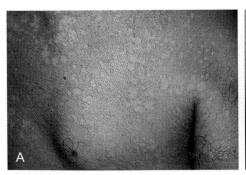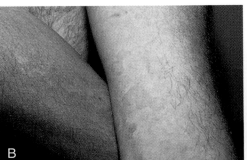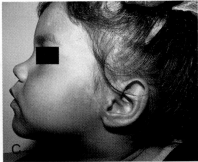

FIGURE 7–32

Tinea versicolor. **A,** Innumerable finely scaly hypopigmented thin papules on the trunk and proximal extremities. **B,** Hypopigmented and hyperpig-mented lesions in the same patient. The lesions on the sun-exposed dor-sal forearms were hypopigmented, whereas those on the relatively sun-protected volar forearms were hyperpigmented compared with normal skin. **C,** Hypopigmented finely scaly papules extending onto the face of a 3-year-old child.

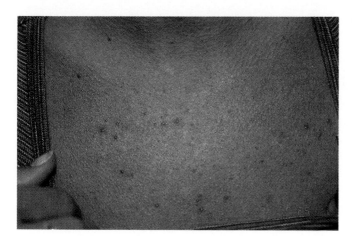

FIGURE 7-33

Pityrosporum folliculitis. Monomorphous pinpoint papulopustules.

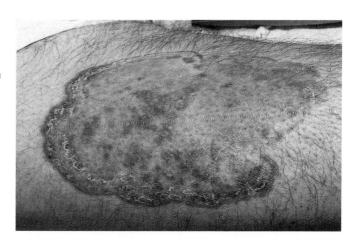

FIGURE 7-34

Tinea corporis on the thigh of a patient with AIDS. Large scaling erythematous plaque with numerous papules within it.

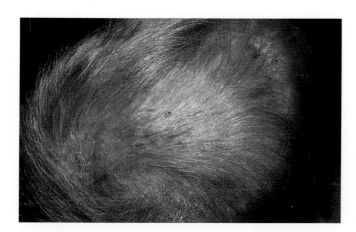

FIGURE 7-35

Tinea capitis in a 6-year-old girl receiving chemotherapy for Wilms tumor.

STAPHYLOCOCCAL AND STREPTOCOCCAL INFECTIONS

Some of the most dramatic skin infections are caused by *Staphylococcus aureus* and *Streptococcus pyogenes.* In addition to skin and soft tissue infections, both organisms have been implicated in the development of toxic shock syndrome. Staphylococcal toxins are also responsible for scalded skin syndrome, which is seen mainly in children.

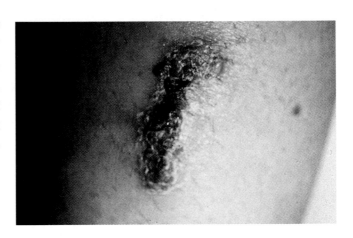

FIGURE 7–36

Impetigo. Infection of the most superficial layer of skin (epidermis) leads to this characteristic infection with a crusty appearance. Topical antibiotics may be all that is necessary for treatment. (Courtesy of Dr. Mark Drapkin, Newton Wellesley Hospital, Newton, Massachusetts.)

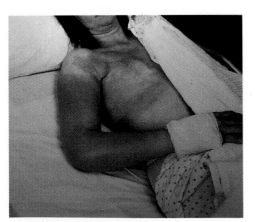

FIGURE 7–37

Erysipelas. After a mastectomy this patient has altered lymphatic drainage in her arm and a superficial infection with *Streptococcus.* The bright red color, edema of the skin, and sharp demarcation suggest erysipelas over cellulitis.

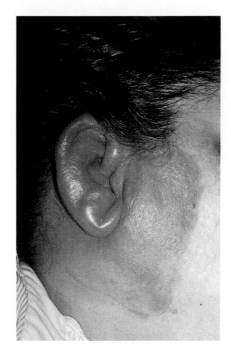

FIGURE 7–38

Erysipelas. Infection on the face is characteristic of erysipelas. Note the sharp borders and the edema, which localize the infection in the superficial dermis.

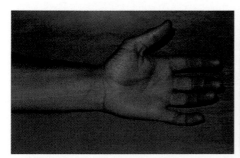 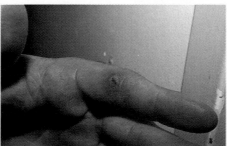 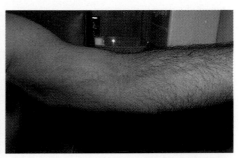

Streptococcal lymphangitis. This superficial infection of the lymphatics is commonly caused by streptococci; however, staphylococci and other organisms including *Erysipelothrix* have also been implicated.

FIGURE 7–39

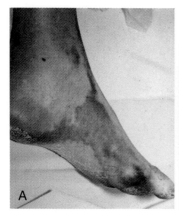
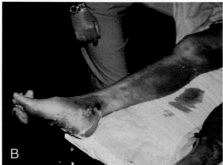
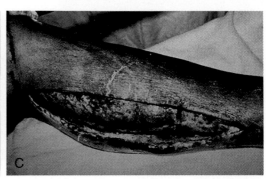

FIGURE 7–40

Streptococcal fasciitis. Infection that extends to the fascia requires surgical debridement of necrotic tissue. The skin becomes discolored because of thrombosis of the blood vessels penetrating through the fascia. The operative specimen in **A** grew group G *Streptococcus.*

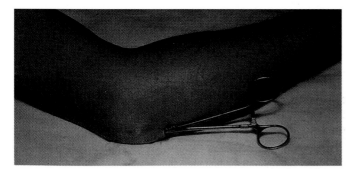

FIGURE 7–41

Streptococcal fasciitis. A Kelly clamp passes beneath the skin without impediment. Counterincisions will be made to plan the extent of the initial debridement.

FIGURE 7–42

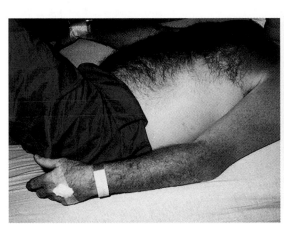

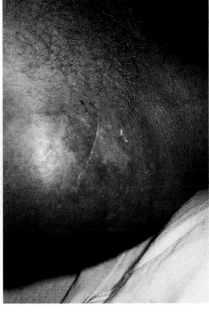

Streptococcal fasciitis. This patient presented with fevers and severe shoulder pain and subsequently grew *Streptococcus intermedius* from the shoulder wound. (Courtesy of Dr. Mark Drapkin, Newton Wellesley Hospital, Newton, Massachusetts.)

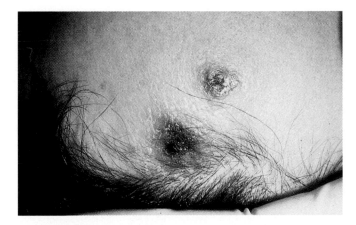

FIGURE 7–43

Ecthyma. *Staphylococcus aureus* was cultured from these embolic lesions. (Courtesy of Dr. Mark Drapkin, Newton Wellesley Hospital, Newton, Massachusetts.)

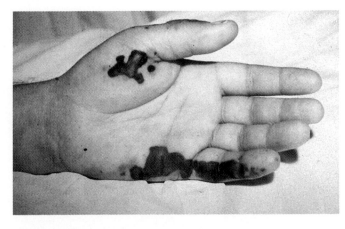

FIGURE 7–44

Necrosis of the skin on the hand following high-grade staphylococcal sepsis.

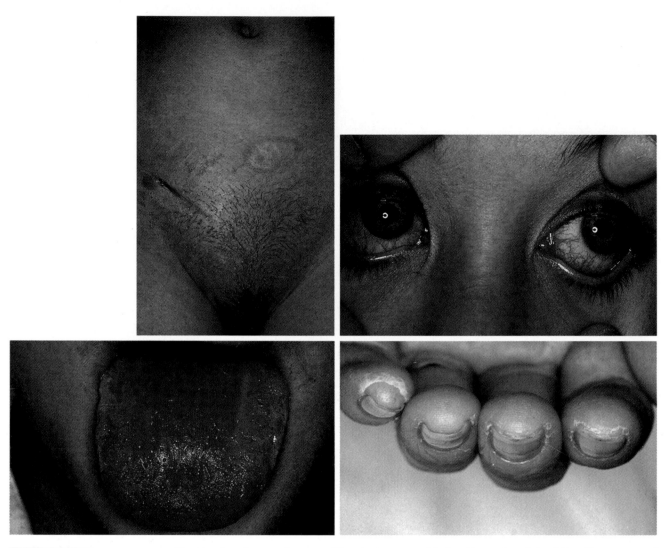

FIGURE 7–45

Toxic shock syndrome. Staphylococcal infection of a tubal ligation wound led to fever and shock associated with conjunctivitis, erythema of the tongue, and desquamation of the fingertips.

FIGURE 7–46

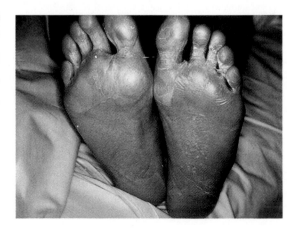

Toxic shock syndrome. Desquamation of the feet is seen in this survivor of toxic shock syndrome. (Courtesy of Dr. Mark Drapkin, Newton Wellesley Hospital, Newton, Massachusetts.)

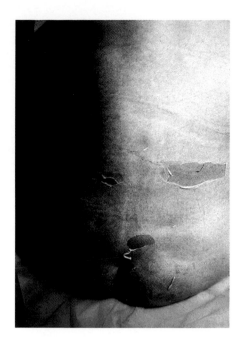

FIGURE 7–47

Scalded skin syndrome. Areas of epidermis are denuded in this infant. This syndrome is caused by an exotoxin produced from *Staphylococcus aureus* phage type 71.

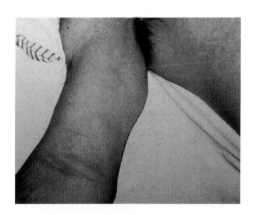

FIGURE 7–48

Scarlet fever. Pastia lines on the arm appear as petechial lesions, which coalesce into linear patterns at pressure sites.

SOFT TISSUE INFECTIONS OF MUSCLE AND FASCIA

Soft tissue infections of fascia and muscle caused by mixed organisms including anaerobes are often fatal if not treated. Early intervention with high doses of antibiotics and radical debridement is necessary. Although such cases are rare, they should all be treated as a medical or surgical emergency. Patients often present with pain in the infected site. Over time, crepitation, edema, skin necrosis, and hemorrhagic bullae appear, and signs of septic shock develop.

TABLE 7–4

Necrotizing Soft Tissue Infections

PARAMETER	GAS-FORMING CELLULITIS	SYNERGISTIC NECROTIZING CELLULITIS	GAS GANGRENE
Predisposing conditions	Traumatic	Diabetes, prior local lesions, perirectal lesions	Traumatic or surgical wound
Incubation period	>3 d	3–14 d	1–4 d
Etiologic organisms	Clostridia, others	Mixed aerobic-anaerobic flora	Clostridia, especially *Clostridium perfringens*
Systemic toxicity	Minimal	Moderate to severe	Severe
Course	Gradual	Acute	Acute
Wound findings			
Local pain	Minimal	Moderate to severe	Severe
Skin appearance	Swollen, minimal discoloration	Erythematous or gangrene	Tense and blanched, yellow-bronze, necrosis with hemorrhagic bullae
Gas	Abundant	Variable	Usually present
Muscle involvement	No	Variable	Myonecrosis
Discharge	Thin, dark, sweetish or foul odor	Dark pus or "dishwater," putrid	Serosanguineous, sweet or foul odor
Gram stain	PMNs, gram-positive bacilli	PMNs, mixed flora	Sparse PMNs, gram-positive bacilli
Surgical therapy	Débridement	Wide filleting incisions	Extensive excision, amputation

PMNs, Polymorphonuclear leukocytes.
From Bartlett JG: Clostridial myonecrosis and other clostridial diseases. *In* Wyngaarden JB, Smith LH Jr, Bennett JC (eds): Cecil Textbook of Medicine, ed 19. Philadelphia, WB Saunders, 1992, p 1679.

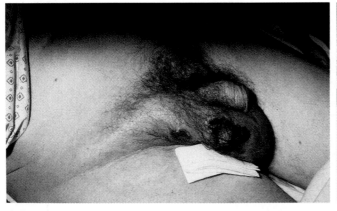
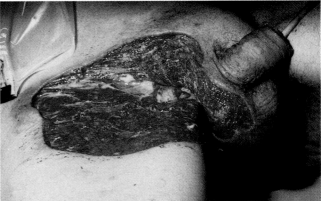

FIGURE 7–49

Fournier gangrene. Necrotizing infection with a mixture of organisms usually starts in the perineum or male scrotum. Careful examination looking for edema and skin necrosis is needed. Debridement along fascial planes is necessary for resolution of the infection. (Courtesy of Dr. Mark Drapkin, Newton Wellesley Hospital, Newton, Massachusetts.)

"STREPTOCOCCAL" MYONECROSIS	NECROTIZING FASCIITIS	INFECTED VASCULAR GANGRENE	STREPTOCOCCAL INFECTION
Trauma, surgery	Diabetes, trauma, surgery, perineal infection	Arterial insufficiency	Traumatic or surgical wound
3–4 d	1–4 d	>5 d	6 h–2 d
Anaerobic streptococci	Mixed aerobic-anaerobic flora	Mixed aerobic-anaerobic flora	*Streptococcus pyogenes*
Minimal until late in course	Moderate to severe	Minimal	Severe
Subacute	Acute to subacute	Subacute	Acute
Late only	Minimal to moderate	Variable	Severe
Erythema or yellow-bronze	Blanched, erythema, necrosis with hemorrhagic bullae	Erythema or necrosis	Erythema, necrosis
Variable	Variable	Variable	No
Myonecrosis	No	Myonecrosis limited to area of vascular insufficiency	No
Seropurulent	Seropurulent or dishwater, putrid	Minimal	None or serosanguineous
PMNs, gram-positive cocci	PMNs, mixed flora	PMNs, mixed flora	PMNs, gram-positive cocci in chains
Excision of necrotic muscle	Wide filleting incisions	Amputation	Débridement of necrotic tissue

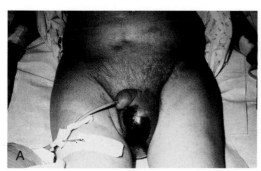
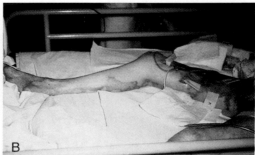
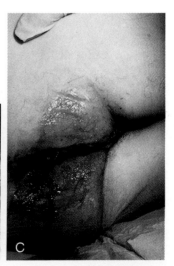

Fournier gangrene. Infection may spread from the scrotum to the anterior abdominal wall **(A)**, the lower leg **(B)**, and the buttocks **(C)**. (Courtesy of Dr. Mark Drapkin, Newton Wellesley Hospital, Newton, Massachusetts.)

FIGURE 7–50

FIGURE 7–51

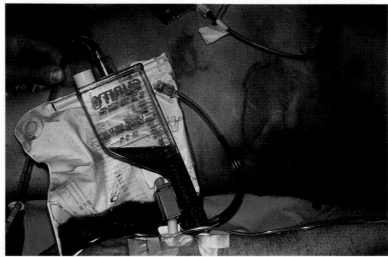

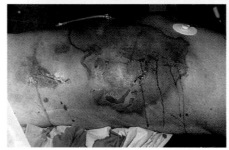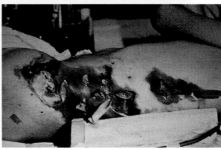

Gas gangrene. *Clostridium perfringens* infection of the abdominal wall following a cholecystectomy and common bile duct exploration. Note the black urine, a sign of massive hemolysis due to liberation of the alpha toxin.

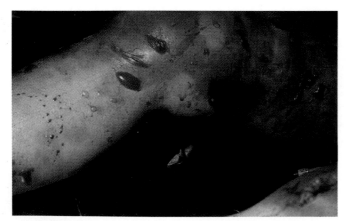

FIGURE 7–52

Gas gangrene. *Clostridium septicum.* Note the discolorations suggestive of skin necrosis. The bullae are characteristic. The fluid is devoid of polymorphonuclear cells. Organisms are easily seen on a Gram stain from bullae fluid or tissue. (Courtesy of Dr. Mark Drapkin, Newton Wellesley Hospital, Newton, Massachusetts.)

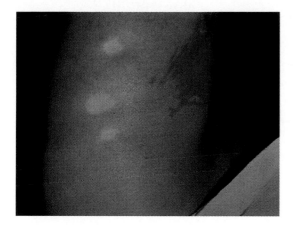

FIGURE 7–53

Fasciitis. Edema of the skin and soft tissue is often present in fasciitis or gas gangrene. Patients will complain of pain in the region, but erythema may not be evident.

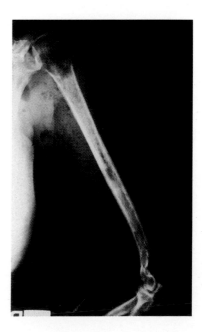

FIGURE 7–54

Gas gangrene. Radiographs are extremely sensitive in picking up gas within tissues even before it can be palpated. This example of gas gangrene reveals extensive disease.

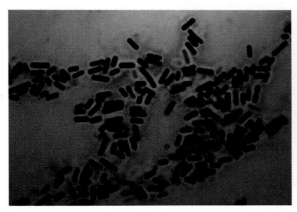 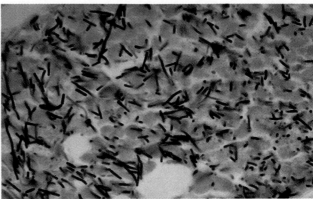

FIGURE 7–55   Clostridial infection. Gram stains show gram-positive rods that look at times like boxcars.

TABLE 7–5

The Most Common Deep Tissue Isolates from 32 Diabetic Patients with Moderate to Severe Foot Infections

MICROORGANISMS ISOLATED	PERCENTAGE OF PATIENTS STUDIED
Aerobes	
Gram-negative bacilli	
Proteus mirabilis	28
Escherichia coli	16
Pseudomonas aeruginosa	16
Enterobacter aerogenes	12
Enterobacter cloacae	6
Citrobacter freundii	6
Gram-positive cocci	
Enterococcus spp.	41
Staphylococcus aureus	25
Group B streptococci	16
Other streptococci	12
Group E nonenterococci	12
Coagulase-negative staphylococci	10
Anaerobes	
Gram-negative bacilli	
Bacteroides fragilis	19
Bacteroides ovatus	9
Bacteroides ureolyticus	9
Prevotella melaninogenica (formerly Bacteroides melaninogenicus)	7
Bacteroides capillosus	7
Gram-positive cocci	
Peptostreptococcus magnus	28
Peptostreptococcus anaerobius	19
Peptostreptococcus asaccharolyticus	9
Gram-positive bacilli	
Clostridium bifermentans	9

Data from Sapico FL, Witte JL, Canawati HN, et al: The infected foot of the diabetic patient: Quantitative microbiology and analysis of clinical features. Rev Infect Dis 6(Suppl 1): 171–176, 1984.

CUTANEOUS MANIFESTATIONS
OF MISCELLANEOUS INFECTIONS

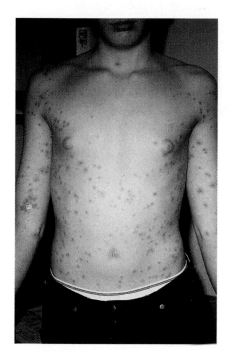

FIGURE 7–56

Pseudomonas. This 16-year-old developed folliculitis following immersion in a hot tub. Cultures of the lesions grew *Pseudomonas aeruginosa.* (Courtesy of Dr. John Cohen, Newton, Massachusetts, and Dr. Mark Drapkin, Newton Wellesley Hospital, Newton, Massachusetts.)

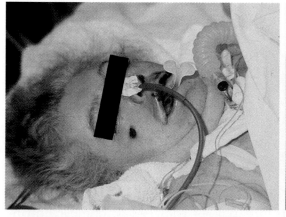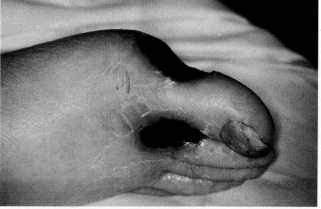

Ecthyma gangrenosum. *Pseudomonas aeruginosa* sepsis with emboli to the skin leading to necrosis. Initially the lesions are round, purple macules with central necrosis. These lesions are often seen in immunocompromised or neutropenic patients undergoing chemotherapy. Cultures of biopsy specimens would reveal the organism.

FIGURE 7–57

FIGURE 7–58

Gram-negative sepsis. Symmetric, peripheral gangrene is caused by disseminated intravascular coagulation in patients with severe sepsis. Gram-negative organisms are often responsible.

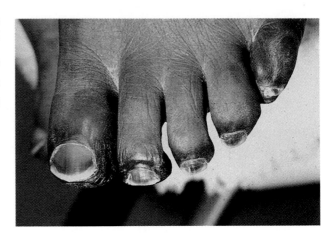

FIGURE 7–59

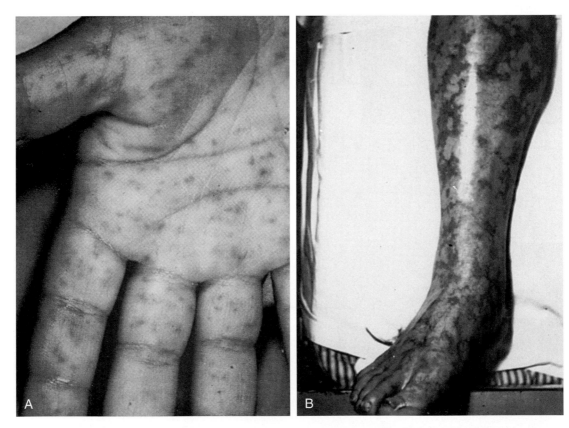

A, Petechial rash on the palm of a patient with Rocky Mountain spotted fever (RMSF). **B,** Purpuric rash in a patient with RMSF complicated by widespread *Rickettsia rickettsii*–mediated vascular injury. (*B* from Woodward TE: Rickettsial diseases in the United States. Med Clin North Am 43: 1516, 1959.)

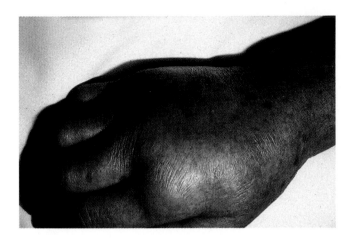

FIGURE 7–60

Pasteurella multocida. Swelling, erythema, and lymphangitis are common after bite wounds from dogs and cats. (Courtesy of Dr. Mark Drapkin, Newton Wellesley Hospital, Newton, Massachusetts.)

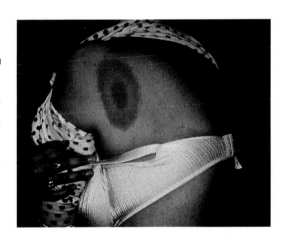

FIGURE 7–61

Lyme disease. Erythema chronicum migrans. Classic target lesion with central clearing is noted. The lesions are cool to the touch. Organisms can be cultured from a biopsy of these lesions. (Courtesy of Dr. Linden Hu, New England Medical Center, Boston, Massachusetts.)

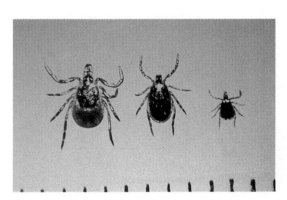

FIGURE 7–62

Deer ticks implicated in the transmission of Lyme disease.

FIGURE 7–63

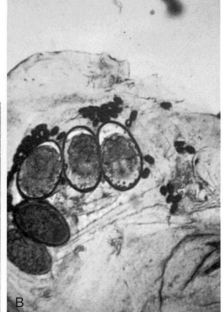

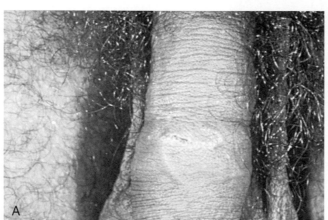

A, Sinuous burrow of scabies mite in a characteristic site. **B,** Eggs and feces of a scabies mite in a skin scraping.

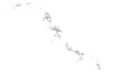

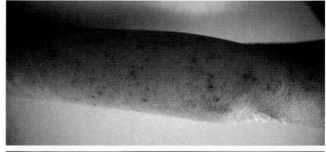

FIGURE 7–64

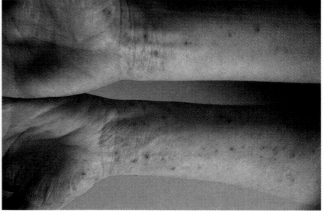

Health care worker who developed scabies from an AIDS patient with Norwegian scabies. Initially the lesions were considered to be a latex allergy.

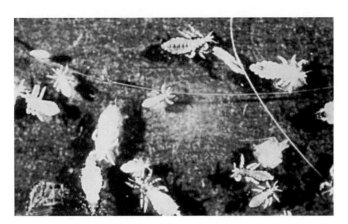

FIGURE 7–65

Body lice and nits concentrated in the seams of clothing. (From Parish LC, Schwartzman RM, Nutting WB [eds]: Cutaneous Infestations of Man and Animals. Copyright © 1983 by Praeger Publishers. Reproduced with permission of Greenwood Publishing Group, Inc., Westport, Connecticut.)

FIGURE 7–66

Pubic lice and nits infesting pubic hairs. (From Domonkos AN, Arnold HL Jr: Diseases of the Skin, ed 7. Philadelphia, WB Saunders, 1982, p 556.)

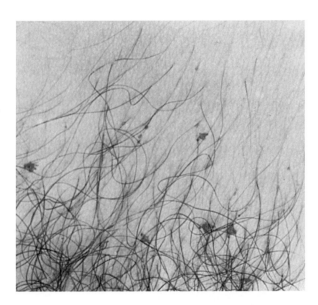

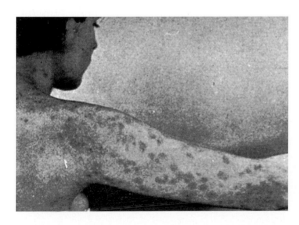

FIGURE 7–67

Macules due to chronic exposure to the bites of body lice. (From Domonkos AN, Arnold HL Jr: Diseases of the Skin, ed 7. Philadelphia, WB Saunders, 1982, p 557.)

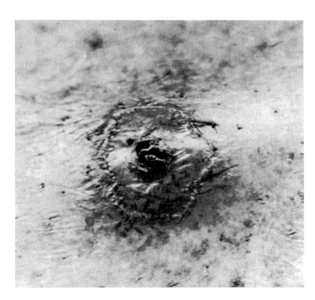

FIGURE 7–68

Furuncular myiasis due to the human botfly. The posterior end of the warble fly *Dermatobia hominis* can be seen, with the shiny black spiracles in the center of the dermal lesion. (Courtesy of the Armed Forces Institute of Pathology. Photograph no. N-49503.)

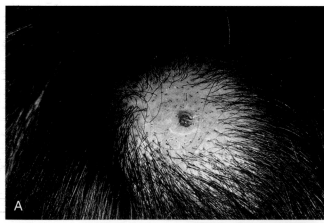

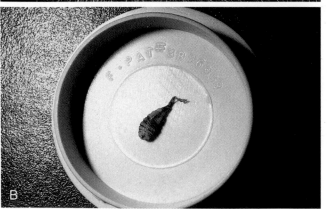

FIGURE 7–69

Myiasis. Ulcerative scalp lesion typical of myiasis. Larvae of *Dermatobia hominis.* (*A* courtesy of Dr. David Hamer, New England Medical Center, Boston, Massachusetts; *B* courtesy of Dr. Mark Drapkin, Newton Wellesley Hospital, Newton, Massachusetts.)

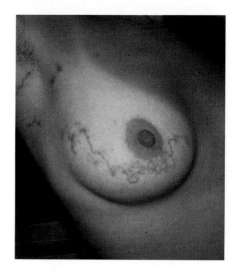

FIGURE 7–70

Cutaneous larva migrans. Filariform larvae from a nonhuman hookworm may persist in the skin for months. This patient had been sun bathing in the tropics.

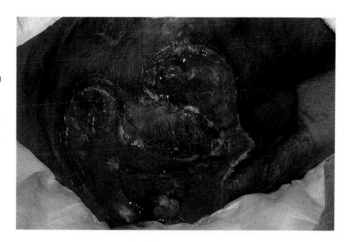

FIGURE 7–71

Decubitus ulcer. This patient with AIDS and paraplegia developed this ulceration over 1 month. Erosion of the hip capsule reveals the femoral head.

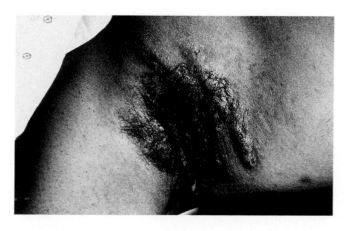

FIGURE 7–72

Hidradenitis suppurativa. Suppurative inflammation of the apocrine glands in the axilla or groin. Bacterial infection is of mixed origin. (Courtesy of Dr. Robert Newton, Newton Wellesley Hospital, Newton, Massachusetts.)

Drug Reactions

Allergic reactions can manifest in multiple ways. Erythroderma and papular or macular rashes are common.

FIGURE 7–73

Toxic epidermal necrolysis. Extensive erosion of skin is noted. This patient recently had been placed on amoxicillin. (Courtesy of Dr. Mark Drapkin, Newton Wellesley Hospital, Newton, Massachusetts.)

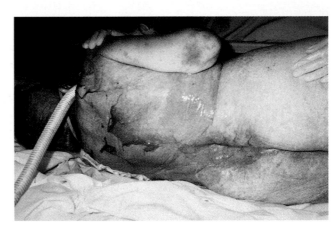

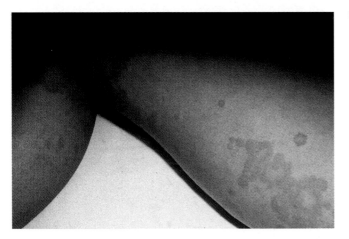

FIGURE 7–74

Erythema multiforme. Drug reaction to minocycline. (Courtesy of Dr. David Hamer, New England Medical Center, Boston, Massachusetts.)

8

INFECTIONS OF THE EYE AND ORBIT

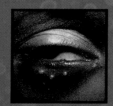 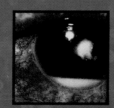 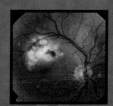

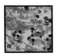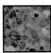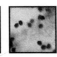

Infections of the eye and orbit have special significance because of the risk of blindness. It is important to assess quickly the location and extent of infection and which organisms most likely are involved. Infections tend to be localized to one compartment (Fig. 8–1), which helps in the management of these infections. Invasive eye infections are medical emergencies that should be treated by experienced clinicians.

FIGURE 8–1

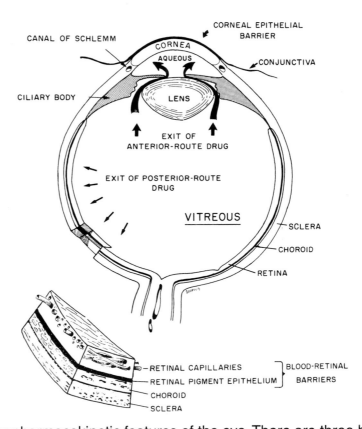

The major pharmacokinetic features of the eye. There are three barriers to ocular penetration: the corneal epithelium, the blood-aqueous barrier (in the ciliary body), and the blood-retinal barriers. The outer blood-retinal barrier is in the retinal pigment epithelium; the inner one lies in the tight junctions of the retinal capillaries. Each contains an active transport pump for organic anions. Anterior-route drugs (aminoglycosides) leave the vitreous by way of the aqueous humor and canal of Schlemm. Posterior-route drugs (penicillins, cephalosporins) leave by active transport across the retina. (From Barza M: Pharmacokinetics of antibiotics. *In* Sabath LD [ed]: Action of Antibiotics in Patients. Bern, Switzerland, Hans Huber, 1982, pp 11–39.)

INFECTIONS IN THE PERIORBITAL REGION

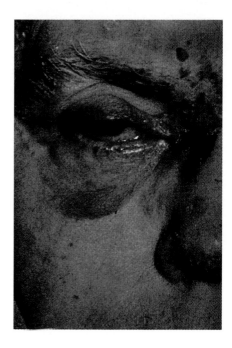

FIGURE 8–2

Varicella zoster. Lesions are in the ophthalmic division of the trigeminal nerve. Slit lamp evaluation is necessary to identify keratitis.

FIGURE 8–3

Molluscum contagiosum. Lesions are seen around the eyes and eyelids. The umbilicated appearance is characteristic. Lesions may be multiple, especially in human immunodeficiency virus (HIV)-positive patients.

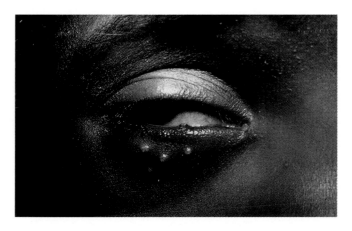

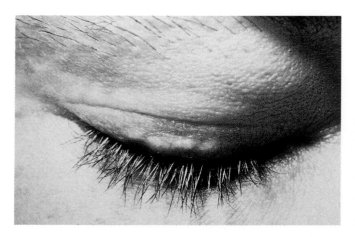

FIGURE 8–4

Loa loa of the eyelid. Migration of the filarial parasite through the subcutaneous tissue is common. At times the worm may migrate across the sclera or conjunctiva.

FIGURE 8–5

Diagram of the lacrimal apparatus. (From Barza M, Baum J: Ocular infections. Med Clin North Am 67: 131–152, 1983.)

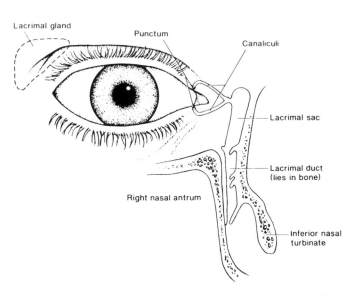

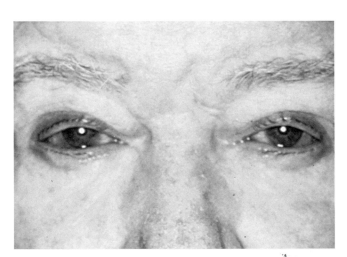

FIGURE 8–6

Staphylococcal blepharitis. Note erythema of lid margins.

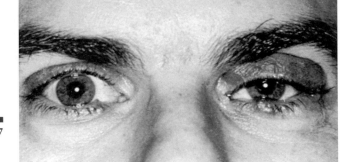

FIGURE 8–7

Multiple bilateral chalazia.

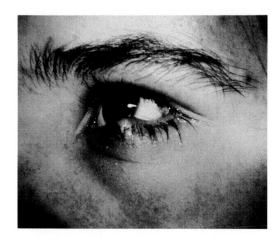

FIGURE 8–8

Hordeolum. The sty is caused by infection of an eyelash follicle or one of the sebaceous or apocrine glands. It can be differentiated from a chalazion, which tends to open into the conjunctival side of the lid.

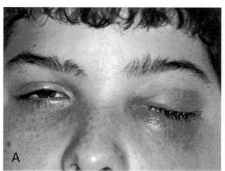 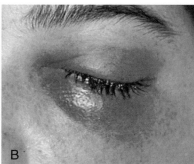 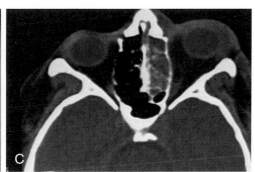

A, and **B,** Orbital cellulitis: patient with left lid swelling, ptosis, and erythema. **C,** CT scan of same patient with left ethmoid sinusitis.

FIGURE 8–9

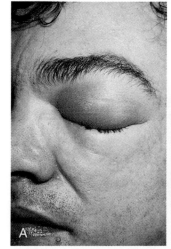 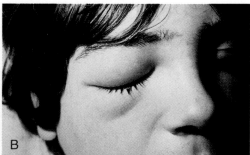 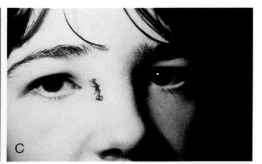

A, Patient with orbital cellulitis caused by *Haemophilus influenzae* group B. Although now rare in the pediatric population, it still needs to be considered in adults. **B** and **C,** Patient with orbital cellulitis that required a medial incision for drainage. Cultures from this patient grew *Streptococcus pneumoniae.* Other organisms frequently responsible are *Staphylococcus aureus* and *Streptococcus pyogenes.* (Courtesy of Dr. Mark Drapkin, Newton Wellesley Hospital, Newton, Massachusetts.)

FIGURE 8–10

TABLE 8–1

Microbiology of Endophthalmitis

ORGANISM	POSTOPERATIVE INFECTIONS (%) (N = 63)	BLEB-ASSOCIATED INFECTIONS (%) (N = 30)	TRAUMATIC INFECTIONS (%) (N = 30)
Staphylococcus epidermidis	38	0	20
Staphylococcus aureus	21	7	0
Streptococcus spp.	11	57	13
Bacillus spp.	0	0	27
Haemophilus influenzae	3	23	0
Other gram-negative species	13	7	20
Fungi	8	3	17
Other	6	3	3
Mixed flora	2	0	11

Modified from Forster RK: Endophthalmitis. *In* Duane TD, Jaeger AE (eds): Clinical Ophthalmology, Vol 4. Philadelphia, Harper & Row, 1994, p 11.

FIGURE 8–11

Two images of bacterial endophthalmitis. Note the appearance of a 5% to 10% hypopyon. (Courtesy of Dr. Jay Duker, New England Medical Center, Boston, Massachusetts.)

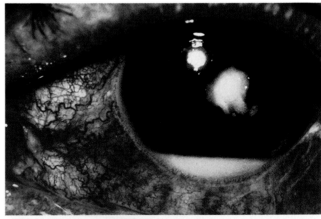
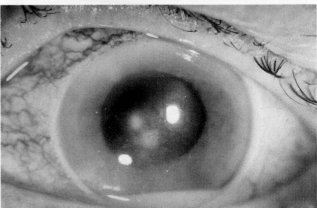

CONJUNCTIVITIS, KERATITIS, AND IRITIS

TABLE 8–2

Features That Distinguish Bacterial from Viral and Chlamydial Conjunctivitis

FEATURE	BACTERIAL CONJUNCTIVITIS	VIRAL CONJUNCTIVITIS	CHLAMYDIAL CONJUNCTIVITIS
Conjunctival injection	Moderately severe	Minimal	Absent or minimal
Exudate	Moderate to profuse (polymorphonuclear)	Minimal (usually mononuclear)	Minimal in adults, copious in newborns
Sticking of lids on awakening	Yes	No	Absent in adults, present in newborns
Papillae (palpebral conjunctiva)	Present	Usually absent	May be present
Follicles (palpebral conjunctiva)	Usually absent	Present	Present in adults, absent in newborns
Preauricular lymphadenopathy	Absent	Present	Present in adults, absent in newborns
Response to antibiotic therapy	Yes	No	Yes
Duration of untreated disease	Up to several weeks	Several weeks	Persistent

Modified from Barza M, Baum J: Ocular infections. Med Clin North Am 67:131–152, 1983.

TABLE 8–3

Features That Distinguish Conjunctivitis from Keratitis or Iritis

FEATURE	CONJUNCTIVITIS	KERATITIS OR IRITIS
Vision	Normal	May be reduced
Pain	Gritty irritation	True pain
Conjunctiva	Diffuse injection	Ciliary flush
Exudate	Minimal to profuse	Usually none
Mattering of lids (dried exudate)	May be present	Absent
Photophobia	Absent	Present
Lacrimation	Usually absent	Present
Pupillary diameter	Normal	Usually small

Modified from Barza M, Baum J: Ocular infections. Med Clin North Am 67:131–152, 1983.

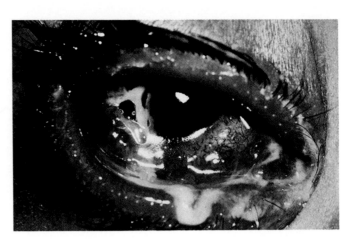

FIGURE 8–12

Bacterial conjunctivitis. Intense inflammation with chemosis of the conjunctivae along with a purulent exudate is noted. Most common organisms include *S. aureus, S. pneumoniae,* and *Neisseria gonorrhoeae.*

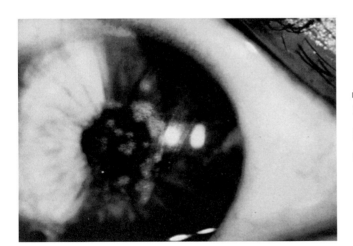

FIGURE 8–13

Subepithelial corneal infiltrates in a patient with epidemic keratoconjunctivitis (adenovirus).

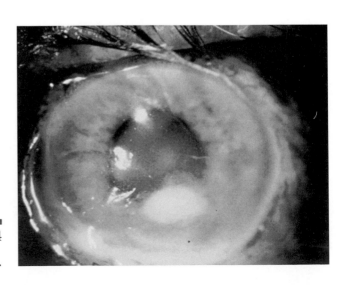

FIGURE 8–14

Bacterial corneal ulcer. Note stromal infiltrate.

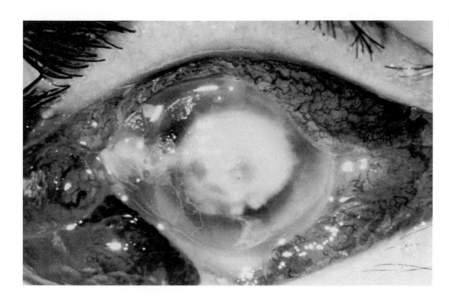

FIGURE 8–15

Fungal ulcer of the cornea. Note satellite lesions.

FIGURE 8–16

Dendritic figures (stained with fluorescein) characteristic of herpes simplex dendritic (epithelial) keratitis.

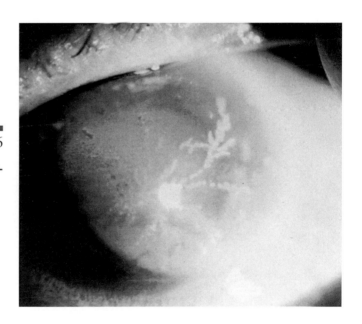

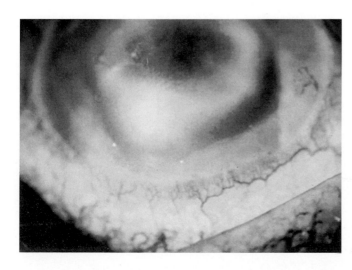

FIGURE 8–17

Acanthamoeba keratitis. Note typical annular appearance with less dense central area.

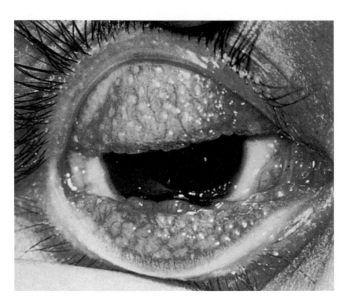

FIGURE 8–18

Severe active trichoma. This stage is characterized by marked follicular reaction and papillary hypertrophy.

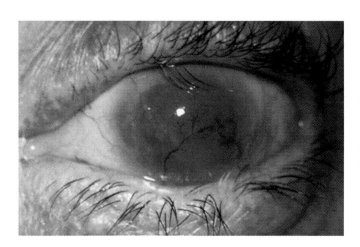

FIGURE 8–19

Trichiasis and entropion in late trachoma. Eyelashes abrade the cornea, ultimately causing a leukoma and blindness.

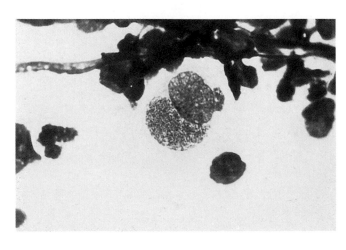

FIGURE 8–20

Chlamydia trachomatis inclusion in a conjunctival smear from a patient with trachoma. Giemsa stain. (Approximately × 1000.)

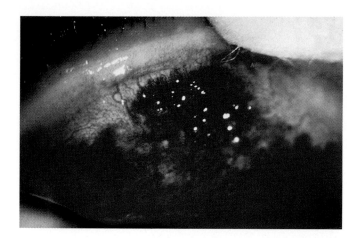

FIGURE 8–21

Kaposi's sarcoma. Lesions on the conjunctiva and eyelid in an HIV-positive patient. (Courtesy of Dr. Jay Duker, New England Medical Center, Boston, Massachusetts.)

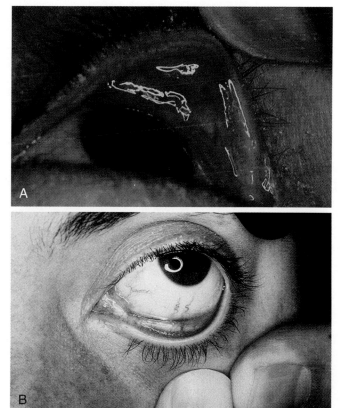

FIGURE 8–22

Endocarditis. Subconjunctival hemorrhage as it appears in these patients is associated with bacterial endocarditis. These findings may be subtle and need to be looked for. (*B* courtesy of Dr. Mark Drapkin, Newton Wellesley Hospital, Newton, Massachusetts.)

INFECTIONS OF THE RETINA

FIGURE 8–23

A, Chorioretinitis caused by *Toxoplasma.* The characteristic lesion is a focal necrotizing retinitis with cottonlike patches in the fundus. Note that the acute lesions *(black arrow)* have indistinct borders and appear soft and white, whereas older lesions *(white arrow)* are whitish gray, sharply outlined, and spotted by accumulations of choroidal pigment. **B,** Toxoplasmic chorioretinitis in a patient with AIDS. (*A* from O'Connor GR: Ocular toxoplasmosis. *In* Locatcher-Khorazo D, Seegal BC [eds]: Microbiology of the Eye. St. Louis, CV Mosby, 1972, p 199; *B* from Polis MA: Differential diagnosis of retinal lesions in persons with HIV infection. Opportunistic Infect Interaction 3:1, 1994.)

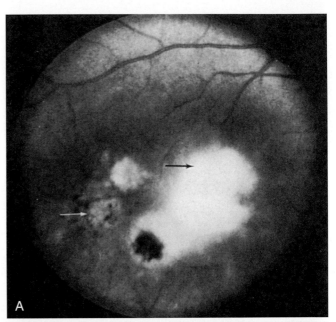

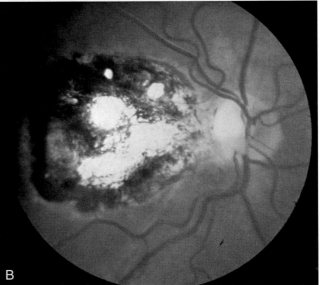

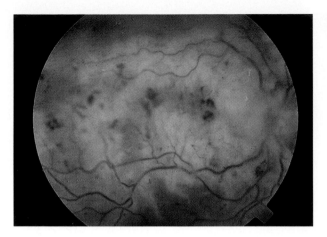

FIGURE 8–24

Acute retinal necrosis due to herpes simplex virus type II. Note extensive swelling of the optic disk and pallor of the retina. Necrosis with hemorrhage is extensive. (Courtesy of Dr. Jay Duker, New England Medical Center, Boston, Massachusetts.)

FIGURE 8–25

HIV retinopathy. Cotton wool spots can be seen as small white patches. These are nerve fiber layer infarcts. (Courtesy of Dr. Jay Duker, New England Medical Center, Boston, Massachusetts.)

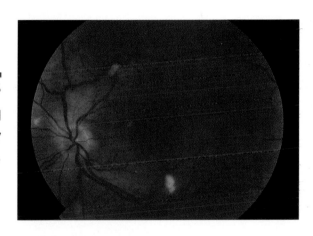

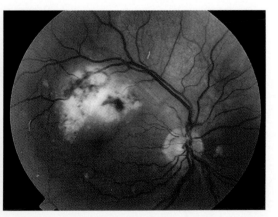

FIGURE 8–26

Cytomegalovirus (CMV) retinitis. Hemorrhage and exudate can be seen in these images of AIDS patients with CMV retinitis. White retinal lesions are seen with hemorrhages and cotton wool spots. (Courtesy of Dr. Jay Duker, New England Medical Center, Boston, Massachusetts.)

FIGURE 8–27

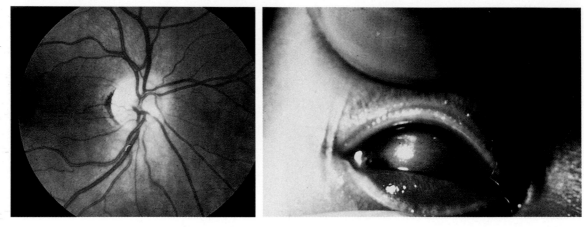

Congenital rubella. Mottled so called salt-and-pepper appearance of the retina. This is due to areas of hyperpigmentation and hypopigmentation of the retina. Other lesions such as cataracts and microphthalmia may also be seen.

FIGURE 8–28

Roth spot. Small areas of hemorrhage are seen in this patient with subacute bacterial endocarditis.

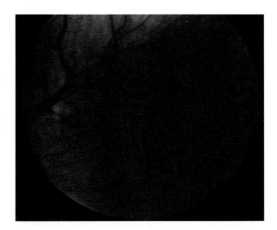

9

INFECTIONS
OF THE
CENTRAL NERVOUS
SYSTEM

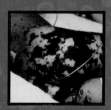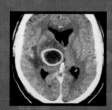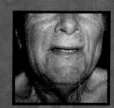

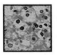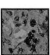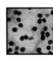

A wide array of microorganisms can infect the central nervous system. It is important to distinguish on clinical grounds infections that are confined to the meninges from those involving the brain. Imaging procedures are helpful in this regard. Some conditions require biopsy or aspiration to make the diagnosis.

MENINGITIS

Meningitis can present as a fulminant infection leading to high morbidity and mortality or it can present in a more insidious manner. Much of this is related to the virulence of the organism and the host response to the infection.

TABLE 9–1

Causative Organisms in Recurrent Meningitis in Adults at Massachusetts General Hospital, 1962 to 1988

ORGANISM	COMMUNITY ACQUIRED (%) (38 EPISODES)	NOSOCOMIAL (%) (41 EPISODES)
Streptococcus pneumoniae	34	2
Gram-negative bacilli*	0	46
Neisseria meningitidis	8	0
Streptococci†	11	2
Staphylococcus aureus	3	15
Haemophilus influenzae	11	0
Mixed bacterial species	0	5
Coagulase-negative staphylococci	0	7
Other	5	2
Culture-negative	29	20

*Exclusive of *H. influenzae.*
†Mainly α-hemolytic, nongroupable strains.
Adapted with permission from Durand ML, Calderwood SB, Weber DJ, et al: Acute bacterial meningitis in adults. A review of 493 episodes. N Engl J Med 328:21–28, 1993. Copyright © 1993 Massachusetts Medical Society. All rights reserved.

TABLE 9–2

Predisposing Factors in Pneumococcal Meningitis*

PREDISPOSING FACTOR	FREQUENCY (%)
Otitis media or mastoiditis†	30
Sinusitis‡	3
Previous head trauma†	10
CSF rhinorrhea§	4
Pneumonia†	20
Neoplastic disease, collagen-vascular disease, or immunosuppression‖	5
Alcoholism‖	9
Diabetes mellitus‖	2

*Compilation from four series of cases occurring between 1956 and 1976.
†Based on data from a total of 459 cases.
‡Based on data from a total of 119 cases.
§Based on data from a total of 281 cases.
‖Based on data from a total of 234 cases.

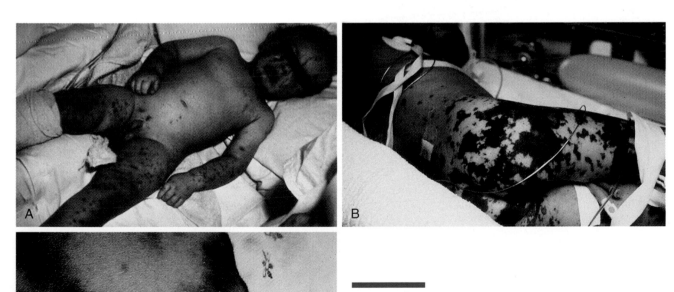

FIGURE 9–1

Purpura fulminans. Patients had meningococcal meningitis and meningococcemia. Coagulopathy leads to the rapid development of these ecchymotic skin lesions. Recognition of such lesions can lead to an early diagnosis of this condition. (Courtesy of W. Hardy Mende III.)

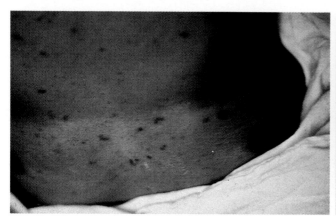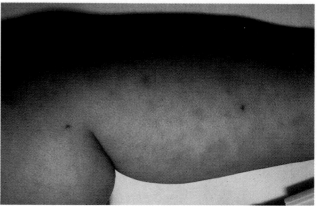

FIGURE 9–2 Skin lesions typical of meningococcemia. Lesions may be mistaken for those due to gonococcemia.

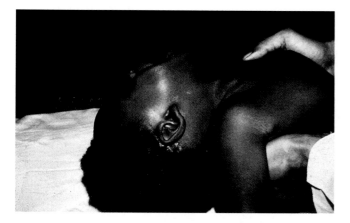

FIGURE 9–3

Meningitis. The nuchal dorsiflexion apparent in this child is produced by meningeal irritation.

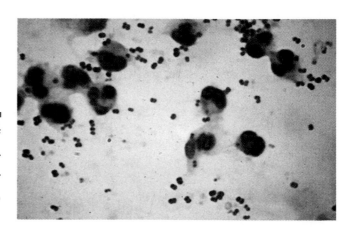

FIGURE 9–4

Meningococci. Cerebrospinal fluid (CSF) from a patient with fulminant meningococcal meningitis. (Courtesy of Dr. Mark Drapkin, Newton Wellesley Hospital, Newton, Massachusetts.)

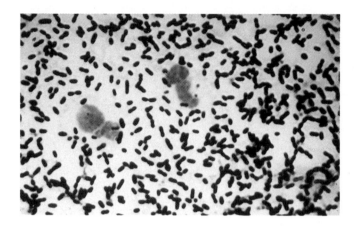

FIGURE 9–5

Pneumococci. CSF from a patient with pneumococcal meningitis.

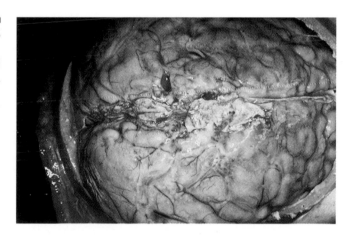

FIGURE 9–6

Purulent meningitis. Brain autopsy specimen showing purulent leptomeninges. This patient died of pneumococcal meningitis. (Courtesy of Dr. Mark Drapkin, Newton Wellesley Hospital, Newton, Massachusetts.)

BRAIN ABSCESS

Computed tomographic (CT) scanning has made diagnosis and treatment of brain abscess much easier. The location of the abscess often suggests the site of origin of the infection. Lesions in the frontal region are associated with sinusitis or orbital spread; lesions in the temporal and parietal regions are often associated with mastoid or middle-ear infections.

TABLE 9–3

Pathogens Most Often Associated with Conditions Occasionally Followed by Brain Abscess*

PREDISPOSING CONDITIONS	PATHOGENS
Otitis, mastoiditis, invaded paranasal sinus, lung abscess, empyema	Usually polymicrobial—anaerobic and microaerophilic streptococci, *Bacteroides, Prevotella, Fusobacterium, Pseudomonas, Proteus* spp., other Enterobacteriaceae†
Noninvaded paranasal sinus, dental	Usually polymicrobial—anaerobic and microaerophilic streptococci, *Bacteroides, Prevotella, Fusobacterium* spp.
Trauma or neurosurgery	Monomicrobial or polymicrobial—*Staphylococcus aureus*, Enterobacteriaceae, *Pseudomonas* spp.
Meningitis (not surgical or traumatic)	*Listeria monocytogenes, Citrobacter diversus*
Bacteremia	
Without apparent source	*Salmonella* spp., *S. aureus, L. monocytogenes*
Genitourinary or gastrointestinal source	Enterobacteriaceae
Wound source	*S. aureus*, Enterobacteriaceae
Endocarditis	Viridans streptococci, enterococci, *S. aureus, Haemophilus aphrophilus, Candida, Aspergillus* spp.

*The extent of the microbiologic evaluation should be dictated by epidemiologic concerns about the potential pathogen. In addition to routine Gram stain and aerobic and anaerobic cultures, prolonged incubation, special media, and evaluation by smear and culture for mycobacteria, fungi, and *Nocardia* organisms may be appropriate for specific patients.
†*Escherichia, Proteus, Klebsiella, Enterobacter, Serratia, Salmonella, Shigella, Arizona, Citrobacter, Edwardsiella, Hafnia, Morganella, Providencia, Yersinia,* and *Erwinia* spp.

TABLE 9–4

Typical Cerebrospinal Fluid Findings in Various Types of Central Nervous System Infections

INFECTION	CELLS/mm³	CELL TYPES*	PROTEIN LEVEL	GLUCOSE LEVEL	CULTURE
Meningitis					
Bacterial	500–10,000	PMNs	High–very high	Low–very low	Positive
Viral	50–1,000	Monocytes	Slightly elevated	Normal	Positive
Tuberculous	50–1,000	Monocytes	High	Low	Positive
Parenchymal					
Brain abscess	5–100	PMNs, monocytes	High–very high	Normal	Negative
Viral encephalitis	5–100	Monocytes	Normal–high	Normal	Negative
Parameningeal					
Epidural	5–100	PMNs, monocytes	High–very high	Normal	Negative
Subdural	5–100	PMNs, monocytes	High	Normal	Negative

*PMNs, Polymorphonuclear leukocytes.

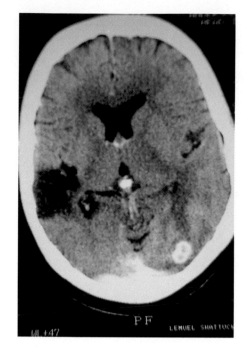

FIGURE 9–7

Staphylococcal brain abscess. Note the bilobed ring enhancement in the right occipital lobe. This patient with endocarditis was an intravenous drug user and had had a remote left middle cerebral artery infarct due to endocarditis 1 year before this CT scan was taken.

FIGURE 9–8

Serial CT scans following therapy for a brain abscess. Note the ring enhancement with vasogenic edema in the right thalamic region, which resolves with therapy.

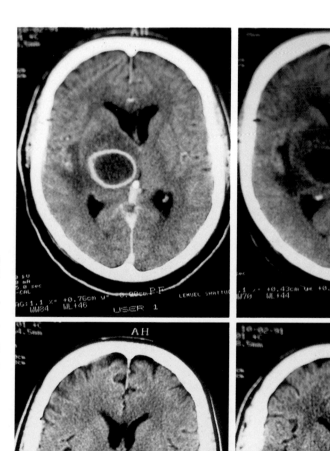

FIGURE 9–9

Tuberculoma. Sagittal view reveals an enhancing lesion in the tectal region of the midbrain. There are also low-signal areas with minimal enhancement in the middle pons. (Courtesy of Dr. Carl Heilman, New England Medical Center, Boston, Massachusetts.)

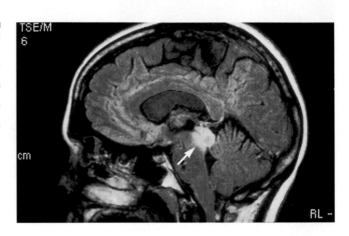

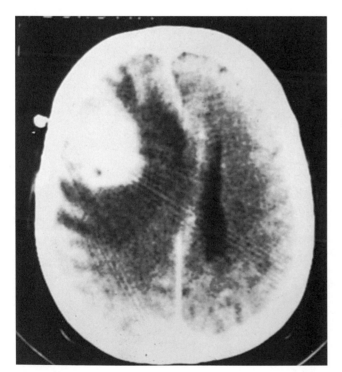

FIGURE 9–10

Computed tomographic scan of the brain shows a large parietal lobe abscess with surrounding edema. (From Bach MC: Nocardial infection. *In* Kass EH, Platt R [eds]: Current Therapy in Infectious Disease—3. Philadelphia, BC Decker, 1990, pp 326–328.)

FIGURE 9–11

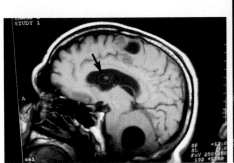
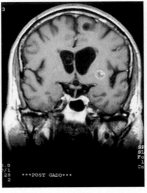
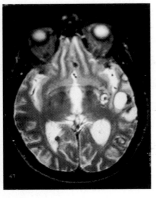

Cysticercosis. Multiple cysticerci are visible in the brain parenchyma and in the ventricles on this magnetic resonance imaging (MRI) scan. Note the protoscolex *(arrow)*. (Courtesy of Dr. Mary Anderson, Lemuel Shattuck Hospital, Boston, Massachusetts.)

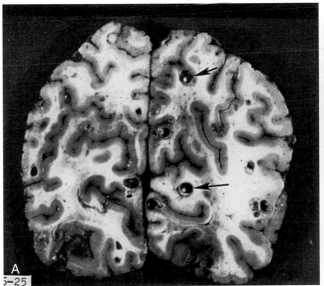
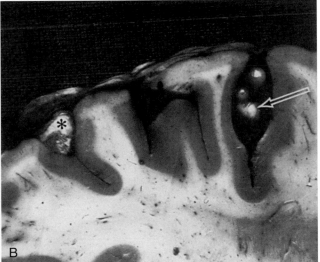

A, Coronal section of human brain showing multiple parenchymatous cysticerci *(arrows)*. **B,** Cortical cysticerci: calcified cyst *(asterisk);* viable cyst *(arrow).* (Courtesy of Dr. Alfonso Escobar Izquierdo, Instituto de Investigaciones Biomédicas, UNAM, Mexico.)

FIGURE 9–12

FIGURE 9–13

A, Cysticercus lodged in aqueduct of fourth ventricle *(arrow).* **B,** *Cysticercus racemosus* in posterior fossa. *Arrows* point to various lobules of this cyst. (Courtesy of Dr. Alfonso Escobar Izquierdo, Instituto de Investigaciones Bìomédìcas, UNAM, Mexico.)

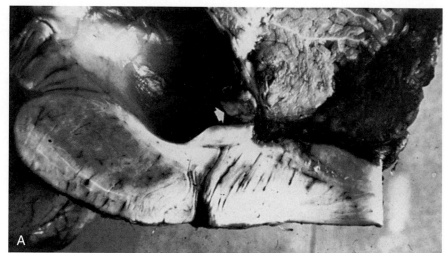

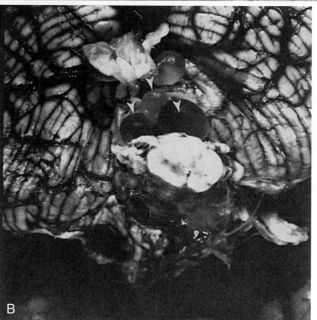

FIGURE 9–14

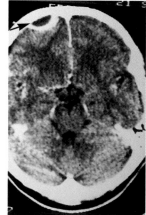

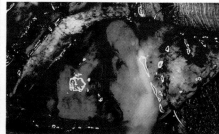

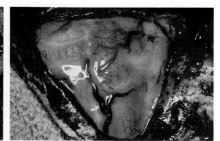

Subdural empyema. Organized area of infection with marked thickening of the meninges *(arrow)* is seen in the frontal lobe of this patient. Exposure of the meninges discloses purulent material. (Courtesy of Dr. Carl Heilman, New England Medical Center, Boston, Massachusetts.)

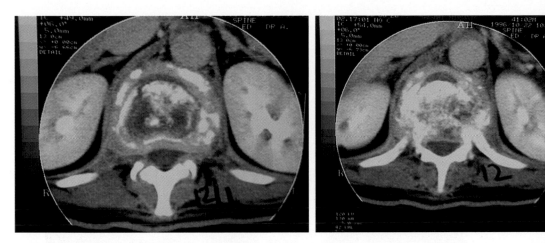

Spinal osteomyelitis with epidural abscess. Anaerobic osteomyelitis with *Bacteroides thetaiotaomicron.* Marked destruction of the vertebral body is due to the chronicity of the infection.

FIGURE 9–15

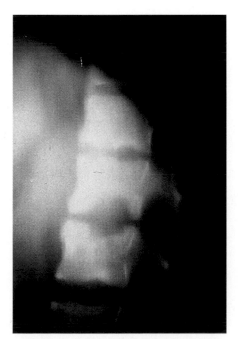

FIGURE 9–16

Spinal osteomyelitis. This tomogram of a child shows bony destruction and disk space narrowing of the lumbar vertebrae.

FIGURE 9–17

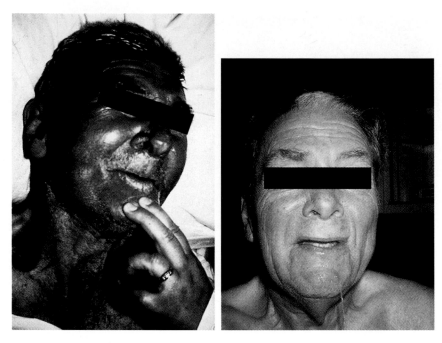

Tetanus. Risus sardonicus—characteristic facies of patients with early stages of tetanus. Difficulty in opening the mouth can be an early clue to the diagnosis of tetanus.

FIGURE 9–18

Gram stain of *Clostridium tetani.* Note the terminal spores.

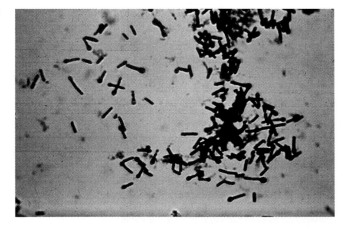

10

MYCOBACTERIAL DISEASES

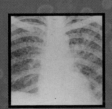
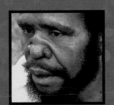
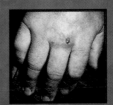

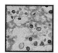

Twenty years ago mycobacterial infections were relatively uncommon in the United States. Recently the incidence of tuberculosis has markedly increased as well as the incidence of disease due to atypical mycobacteria. The reasons for the increased occurrence of mycobacterial infection include increased world travel, increased homelessness, and the rise of human immunodeficiency virus (HIV).

MYCOBACTERIUM TUBERCULOSIS

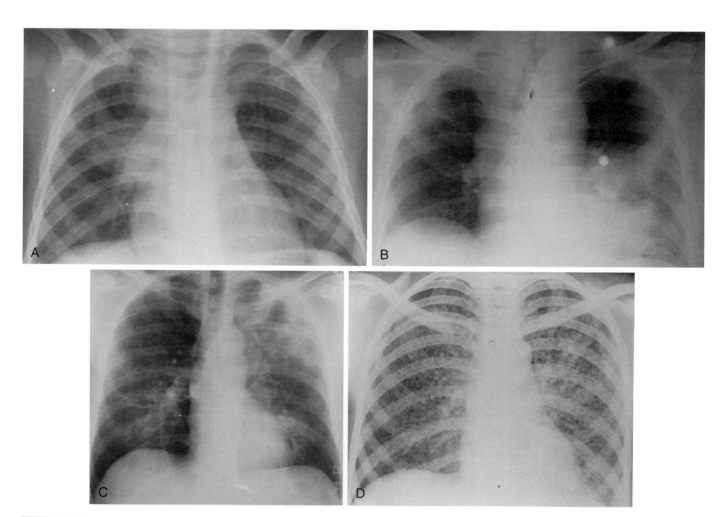

FIGURE 10–1

Chest radiographs of different presentations of tuberculosis. **A,** Primary tuberculosis in a child. (Note right-sided hilar adenopathy, right-sided lower lobe infiltrates, and volume loss.) **B,** Lower lung field tuberculosis infiltration and cavity with air-fluid level in lingula. **C,** Reactivated tuberculosis, far-advanced disease with bronchogenic spread. **D,** Miliary tuberculosis.

FIGURE 10–2

Surgical view of a patient with tuberculosis peritonitis. The multiple tubercles can be seen on the intestinal serosa and on the root of the mesentery.

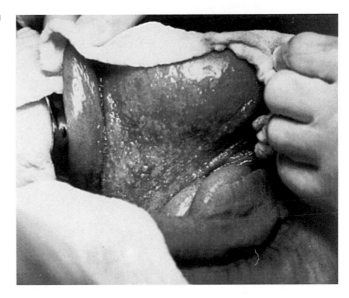

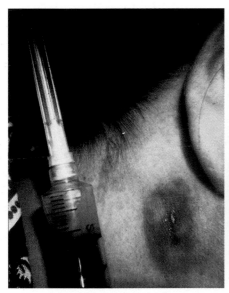

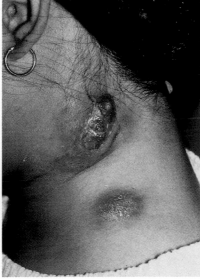

FIGURE 10–3

Cervical tuberculosis. Culture of purulent material grew *M. tuberculosis.*

FIGURE 10–4

Tuberculoma. Small paramedian lesion in the superior left frontal lobe with surrounding vasogenic edema is clearly visible.

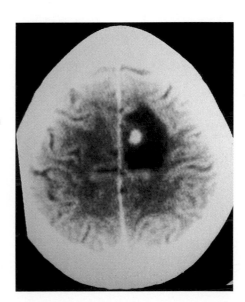

FIGURE 10–5

These dermal lesions developed in an elderly patient with pulmonary tuberculosis. Biopsy revealed *M. tuberculosis.*

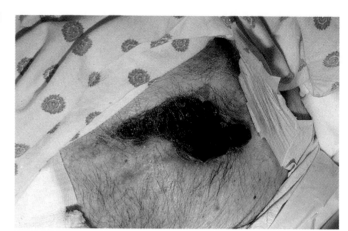

FIGURE 10–6

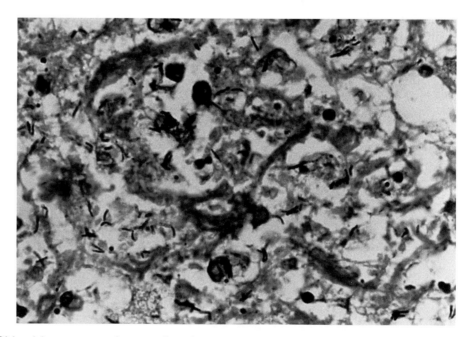

Skin biopsy specimen showing numerous intracellular acid-fast bacilli clumping into globi. (Wade-Fite stain, × 1000.)

MYCOBACTERIUM LEPRAE

TABLE 10–1

Major Histologic and Immunologic Features of the Disease Spectrum in Leprosy*

CHARACTERISTICS	TT	BT	BB	BL	LL
Histologic and Microbial					
Epithelioid cells, mature	++	±	–	–	–
Epithelioid cells, immature	+	++	++	±/–	–
Langhans giant cells, large	++	±/–	–	–	–
Macrophages	–	–	±	++	++
Lymphocytes	+/±	++/±	±	++	±
Bacterial index	0	0–2	3–4	4–5	5–6+
Bacilli in nasal smears	–	–	–	±	++
Immunologic					
Lepromin, Fernandez reaction	++/–	++/–	+/–	–	–
Lepromin, Mitsuda reaction	++/±	++/+	–	–	–
LTT, percent lymphocyte transformation	10	5.7	2.0	0.4	0.2
Antibody, anti–*M. leprae*	–/+	–/++	++	+++	+++

*TT, Tuberculoid leprosy; BT, borderline tuberculoid leprosy; BB, borderline leprosy; BL, borderline lepromatous leprosy; LL, lepromatous leprosy; LTT, lymphocyte transformation test; +++, strongly positive; +, positive; ±, indeterminate; –, negative.

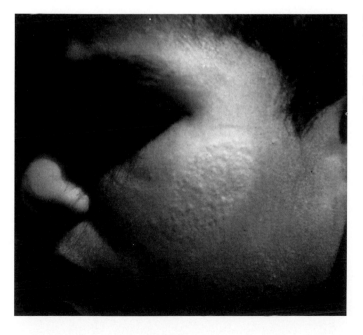

FIGURE 10–7

Tuberculoid skin lesion. This young boy has a single, well-defined anesthetic hypopigmented patch on his cheek.

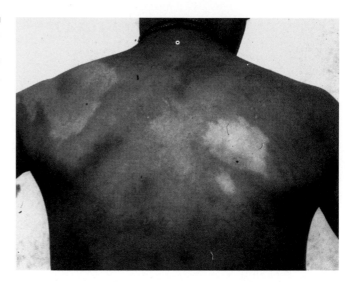

FIGURE 10–8

Borderline tuberculoid skin lesion. This patient has several large, hypopigmented anesthetic skin lesions; satellite lesions are also visible.

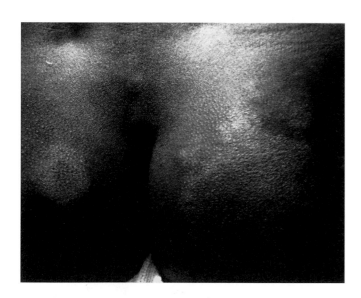

FIGURE 10–9

Borderline leprosy lesion. Numerous skin lesions of all sizes are seen, some with healing centers on this patient's back and buttocks.

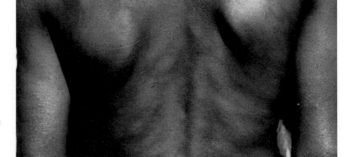

FIGURE 10–10

Multiple ill-defined lesions typical of borderline lepromatous leprosy are present on this patient's back.

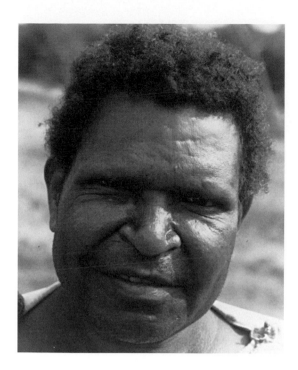

FIGURE 10–11

Moderately advanced lepromatous leprosy. There is symmetric infiltration of the face with particular involvement of the eyebrows, nose, and cheek creases. Eyebrow loss (madarosis) is also present.

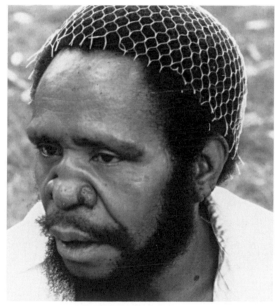

FIGURE 10–12

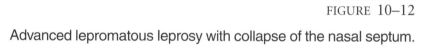

Advanced lepromatous leprosy with collapse of the nasal septum.

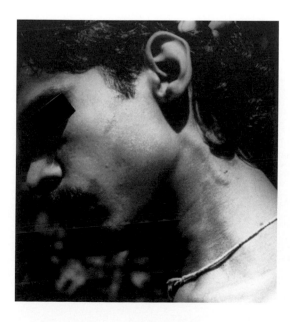

FIGURE 10–13

Visible thickening of the great auricular nerve.

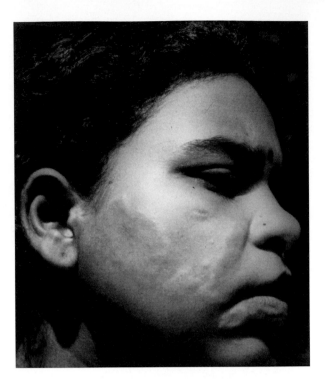

FIGURE 10–14

Reversal reaction lesions. This woman with borderline lepromatous leprosy suddenly developed erythema and edema of her previously quiescent facial lesions 6 weeks after delivery.

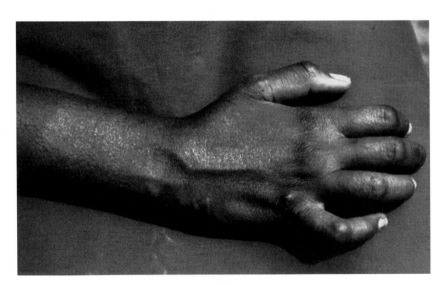

FIGURE 10–15

Reversal reaction acute neuritis. The hand is swollen with clawing of the fingers, indicating involvement of both the ulnar and median nerves.

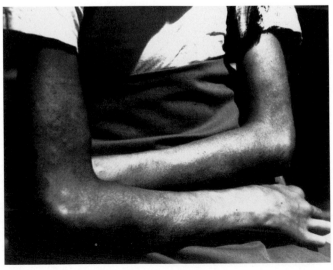

FIGURE 10–16

Typical cutaneous lesions of erythema nodosum leprosum (ENL).

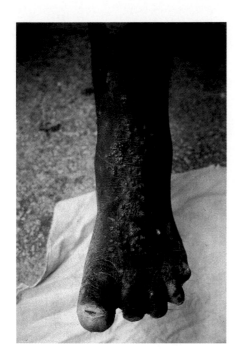

FIGURE 10–17

Deformity and digital atrophy in a patient with leprosy.

ATYPICAL *MYCOBACTERIUM*

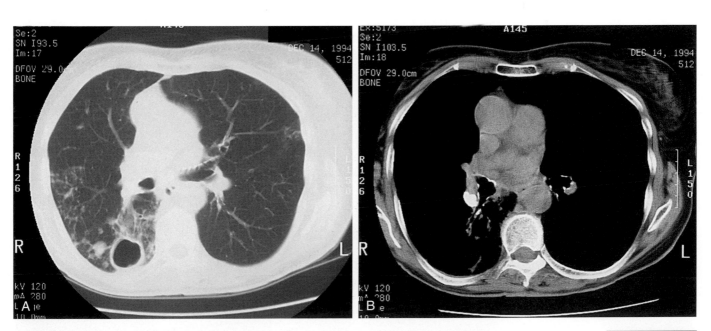

A, A computed tomographic scan in a 75-year-old woman demonstrates cavitary disease in the superior segment of the right lower lobe; sputum cultures repeatedly yielded heavy growth of *Mycobacterium avium* complex (MAC). **B,** The "mediastinal window" at this level demonstrates a large calcified peribronchial lymph node compressing this segmental bronchus. The patient grew up in Illinois, an area in which *Histoplasma capsulatum* is indigenous. Large calcified lymph nodes like this are seen almost exclusively in persons from this region. We believe that prior histoplasmosis predisposes to pulmonary MAC by local lung or bronchial damage.

FIGURE 10–18

FIGURE 10–19

A computed tomographic lung scan of a 43-year-old woman, a nonsmoker, with cystic-saccular bronchiectasis associated with MAC involving the inferior segment of the lingula, abutting the heart, and, to a lesser extent, the medial segment of the right middle lobe, also abutting the heart. This pattern, lingular and middle lobe focal bronchiectasis, is virtually pathognomonic of mycobacterial disease in our experience. In addition, this patient had mild scoliosis, pectus excavatum, and mitral valve prolapse.

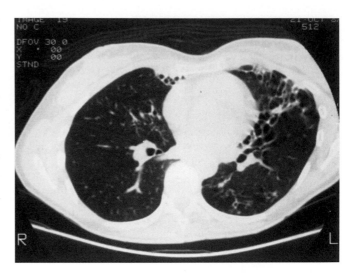

FIGURE 10–20

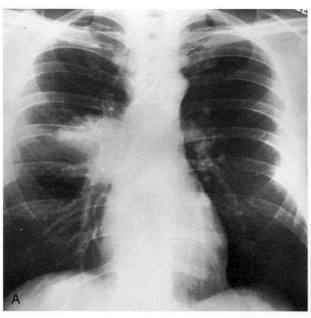
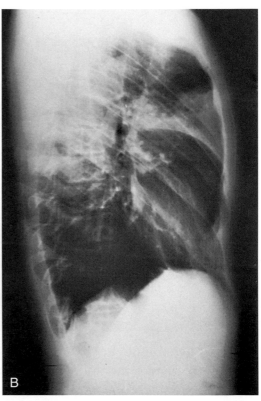

Frontal **(A)** and lateral **(B)** chest radiographs show an infiltration in the anterior segment of the right upper lobe caused by MAC.

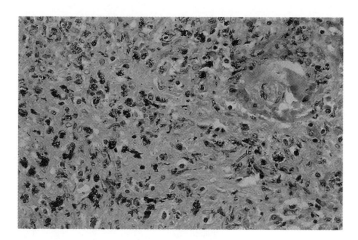

FIGURE 10–21

Mycobacterium avium complex. Autopsy specimen of spleen in a patient with AIDS. Note the extensive burden of organisms seen in this slide.

FIGURE 10–22

Mycobacterium scrofulaceum. Cervical lymphadenitis and drainage caused by atypical mycobacteria.

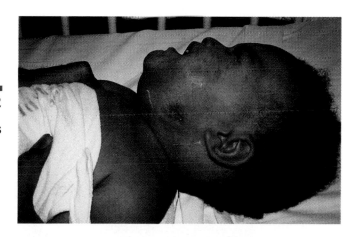

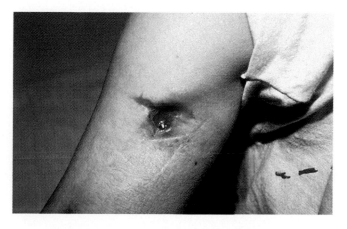

FIGURE 10–23

Mycobacterium haemophilum. Skin lesions developed in a 43-year-old AIDS patient. Lesions resolved with antituberculosis medications.

FIGURE 10–24

Mycobacterium marinum. Nodular lesion developed after abrasion with a marlin fin.

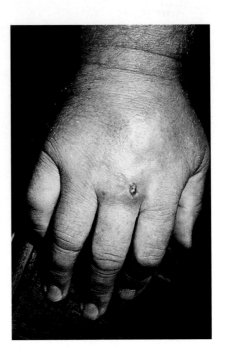

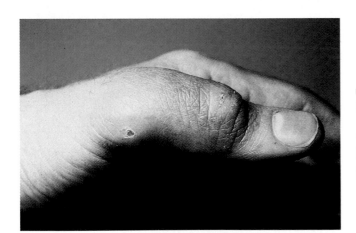

FIGURE 10–25

M. marinum. Lesion developed after hand immersion in an aquarium. (Courtesy of Dr. Mark Drapkin, Newton Wellesley Hospital, Newton, Massachusetts.)

11

VIRAL DISEASES

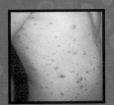

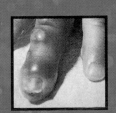

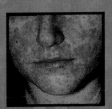

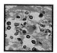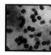

The correct diagnosis of viral exanthems is necessary both for potential drug treatment and public health quarantine.

HERPES VIRUSES

FIGURE 11–1

Schema for the pathogenesis of varicella. It is assumed to involve a biphasic course during the incubation period consisting of a primary and secondary viremia before appearance of the exanthem. (From Grose C: Variation on a theme by Fenner: The pathogenesis of chickenpox. Pediatrics 68:735–737, 1981. Reproduced by permission of Pediatrics.)

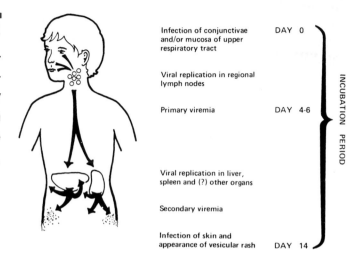

Infection of conjunctivae and/or mucosa of upper respiratory tract	DAY 0
Viral replication in regional lymph nodes	
Primary viremia	DAY 4-6
Viral replication in liver, spleen and (?) other organs	
Secondary viremia	
Infection of skin and appearance of vesicular rash	DAY 14

INCUBATION PERIOD

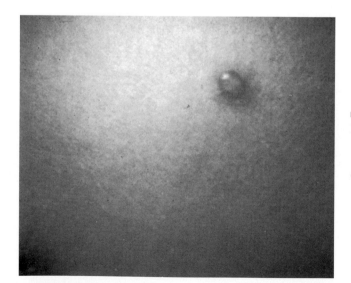

FIGURE 11–2

Initial vesicular lesion of varicella, appearing as a dewdrop on a rose petal.

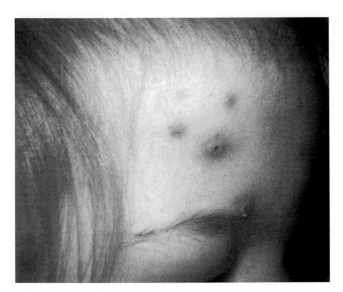

FIGURE 11–3

Vesiculopustular lesions of varicella.

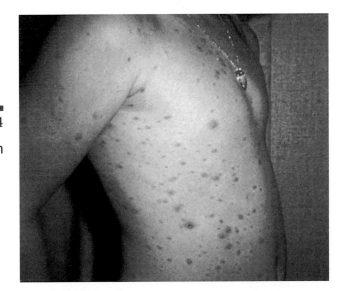

FIGURE 11–4

Varicella, day 2; note truncal distribution and lesions in multiple stages of development.

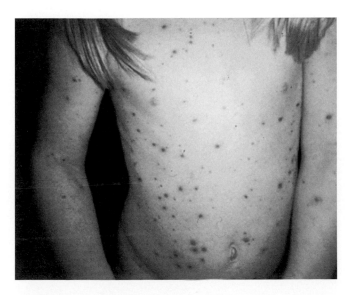

FIGURE 11–5

Varicella, day 4; note crusting of lesions in the same patient as in Figure 11–4.

FIGURE 11–6

Varicella. Hemorrhagic lesions are seen in patients with underlying thrombocytopenia.

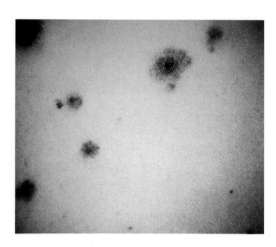

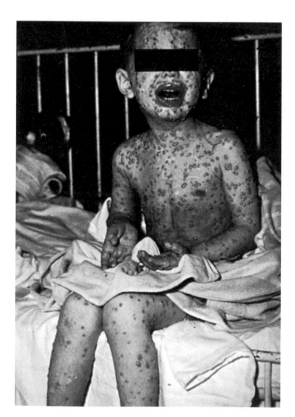

FIGURE 11–7

Disseminated varicella in child with leukemia receiving chemotherapy in 1950s. (Courtesy of Dr. Thomas Weller, Harvard University School of Public Health, Boston, Massachusetts.)

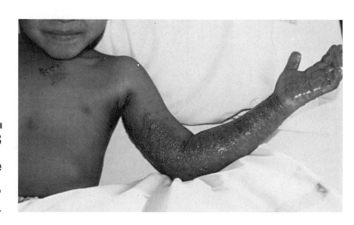

FIGURE 11–8

Herpes zoster in an otherwise healthy child. Note the dermatomal distribution of this unusually severe form, which required skin grafts to restore full range of motion.

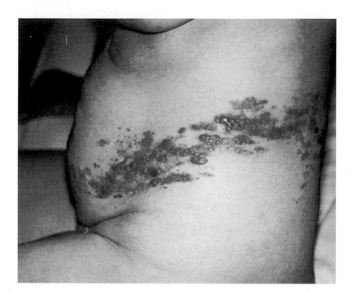

FIGURE 11–9

Herpes zoster in immunosuppressed adult, day 3.

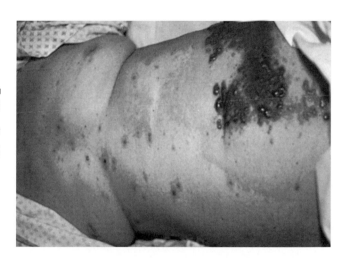

FIGURE 11–10

Herpes zoster in same patient as in Figure 11–9, day 8; note cutaneous dissemination of vesicular rash and hemorrhage into dermatomal lesion.

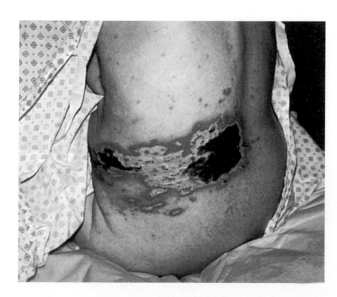

FIGURE 11–11

Herpes zoster in same patient as in Figures 11–9 and 11–10, day 18. Note necrosis and scarring of skin of this person, who developed postherpetic neuralgia.

FIGURE 11–12

A positive rapid varicella zoster virus (VZV) antigen test. Human cells infected with VZV were dried on a glass slide. The cells were covered with a VZV-specific monoclonal antibody tagged with fluorescein. Bright surface staining is easily seen on several cells. Because the VZV rapid antigen test is more sensitive and specific, it should replace the Tzanck test.

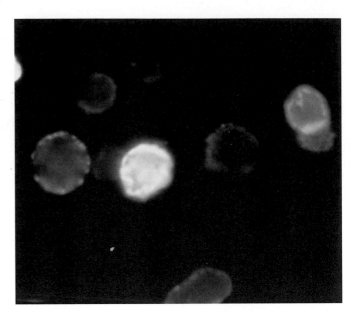

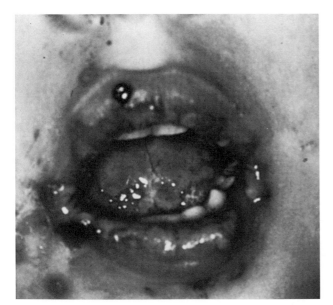

FIGURE 11–13

Acute herpetic gingivostomatitis. In addition to having vesicles on the oral mucosa, palate, and tongue, this child with acute herpetic gingivostomatitis has herpetic vesicles on the lips and perioral skin. (From Oxman MN: Herpes stomatitis. *In* Braude AI, Davis CE, Fierer J [eds]: Infectious Diseases and Medical Microbiology, ed 2. Philadelphia, WB Saunders, 1986, pp 752–772.)

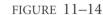

FIGURE 11–14

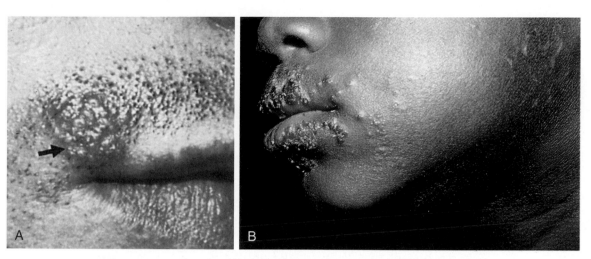

Herpes labialis. After a 12-hour prodrome of localized itching and burning, this medical student developed a small group of erythematous papules that quickly evolved into a typical cluster of vesicles *(arrow)* on an erythematous base. (*A* from Oxman MN: Herpes stomatitis. *In* Braude AI, Davis CE, Fierer J [eds]: Infectious Diseases and Medical Microbiology, ed 2. Philadelphia, WB Saunders, 1986, pp 752–772.)

FIGURE 11–15

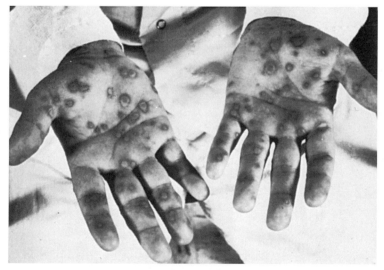

Recurrent erythema multiforme associated with recurrent herpes simplex. A young man with recurrent herpes simplex involving a small area of skin over his left scapula (herpes gladiatorum) regularly develops erythema multiforme 3 to 5 days after the onset of each herpetic recurrence. The rash consists of characteristic target (iris) lesions and involves primarily the skin of the trunk and extremities, including the palms and soles. HSV-1 is regularly isolated from the herpetic lesions over the scapula but not from the target lesions, and no multinucleated giant cells or intranuclear inclusion bodies have been detected in biopsy specimens of the erythema multiforme lesions. (From Oxman MN: Herpes stomatitis. *In* Braude AI, Davis CE, Fierer J [eds]: Infectious Diseases and Medical Microbiology, ed 2. Philadelphia, WB Saunders, 1986, pp 752–772.)

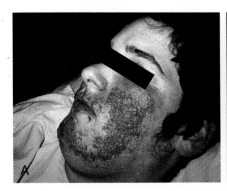
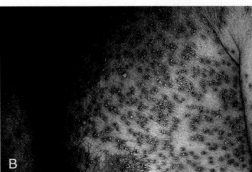
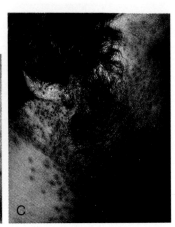

FIGURE 11–16

Eczema herpeticum. Widespread eruptions present in patients with atopic dermatitis. This is often the initial presentation of herpes simplex infection; however, recurrent disease may produce similar widespread lesions. The patient in **C** had superinfection with *Staphylococcus aureus*. (*C* courtesy of Dr. Mark Drapkin, Newton Wellesley Hospital, Newton, Massachusetts.)

FIGURE 11–17

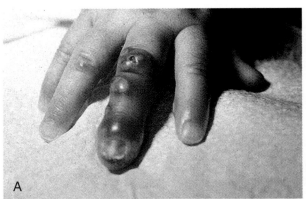
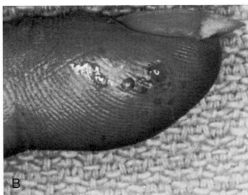

Herpetic whitlow. **A,** Extensive disease is present in this finger. This is often mistaken for bacterial cellulitis. **B,** The terminal phalanx of the index finger of a respiratory therapist is exquisitely painful, swollen, and erythematous, with multiple deep and superficial vesicles. HSV-1 was isolated from vesicle fluid. (*A* courtesy of Dr. Mark Drapkin, Newton Wellesley Hospital, Newton, Massachusetts. *B* from Oxman MN: Herpes stomatitis. *In* Braude AI, Davis CE, Fierer J [eds]: Infectious Diseases and Medical Microbiology, ed 2. Philadelphia, WB Saunders, 1986, pp 752–772.)

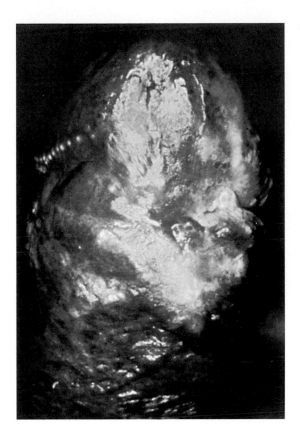

FIGURE 11–18

Cytomegalovirus (CMV) infection. This nondescript penile ulceration was due to cutaneous CMV infection. Biopsy and cultures are necessary to establish this diagnosis.

VIRAL INFECTIONS

FIGURE 11–19

Periungual warts result in nail dystrophy.

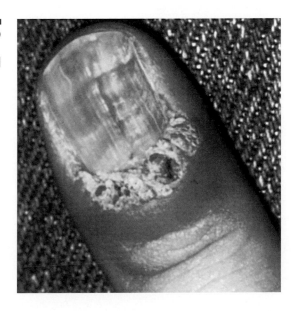

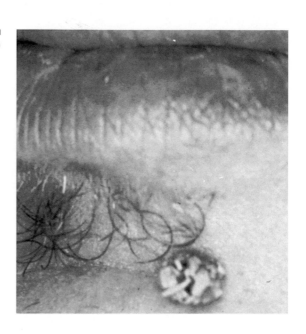

FIGURE 11–20

Filiform warts on the chin.

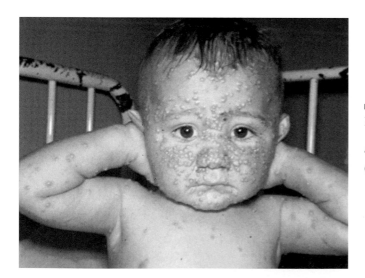

FIGURE 11–21

Appearance of the rash of smallpox on day 6 to 7. All of the lesions are in the same stage of development.

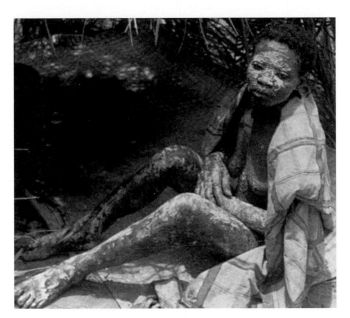

FIGURE 11–22

Denuded areas of skin produced by the sloughing of confluent smallpox lesions.

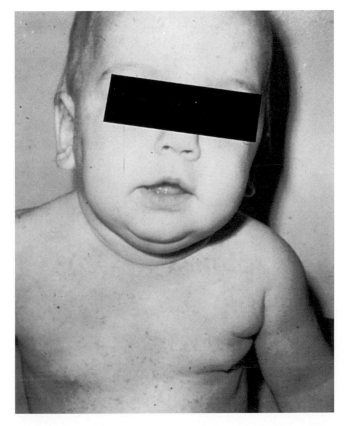

FIGURE 11–23

The scattered maculopapular rash of roseola is most evident on the trunk, the face being relatively spared.

FIGURE 11–24

A lacy or reticular pattern of erythema, as evident on the thigh, is characteristic of erythema infectiosum.

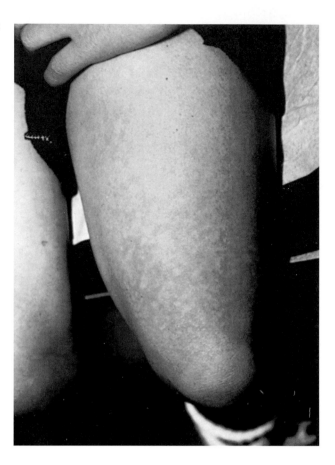

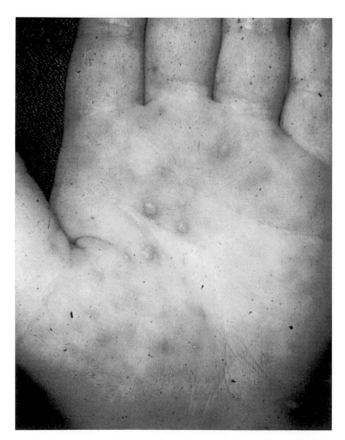

FIGURE 11–25

Multiple vesicles of hand-foot-and-mouth disease are present on the palm.

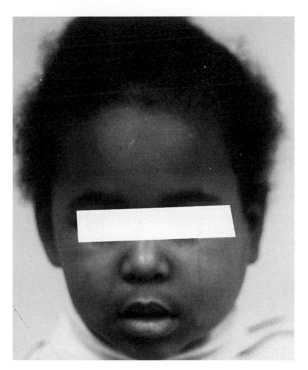

FIGURE 11–26

Female patient with swelling of left parotid gland due to parotitis. Note the difference with the right parotid gland. (Courtesy of Dr. A. Deveikis, Memorial Miller Children's Hospital and Health System, Long Beach, California.)

FIGURE 11–27

Mumps. Swelling of the parotid glands is clearly visible. Orchitis is associated with mumps.

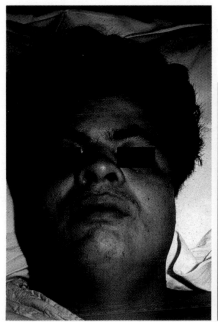
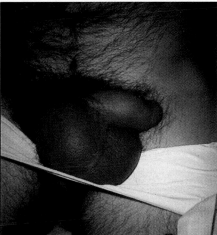

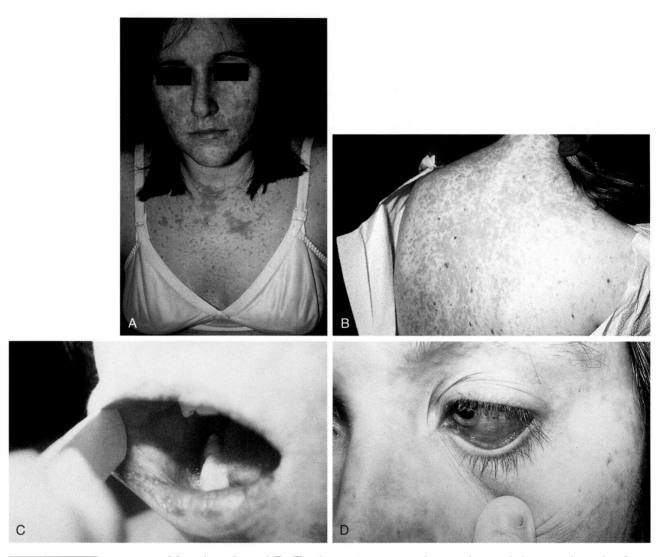

FIGURE 11–28

Measles. **A** and **B,** Erythematous maculopapular rash is noted on the face and neck and trunk. Over time the rash will spread down the extremities. **C,** Koplik spots present on the buccal mucosa. They appear red with small blue-white centers. **D,** Conjunctivitis associated with measles.

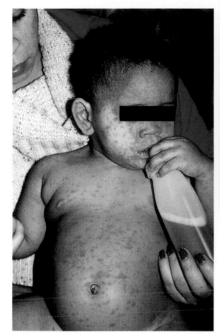

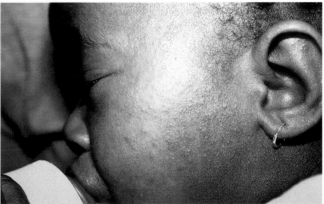

FIGURE 11–29

Infants with measles.

FIGURE 11–30

Close up of skin lesions associated with measles.

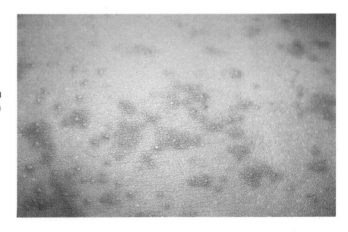

FIGURE 11–31

Kaposi's varicelliform eruption, which is seen mainly in patients with atopic dermatitis who have been immunized with vaccinia virus. Incidence of this infection has been greatly reduced now that immunization is not widespread.

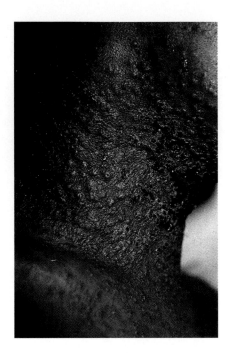

INDEX

Note: Page numbers followed by t refer to tables.